Adolescent Medicine

Controversies and Conundrums

Guest Editors:

Susan M. Coupey, M.D.

Professor of Pediatrics
Albert Einstein College of Medicine
Associate Director, Division of Adolescent Medicine
Montefiore Medical Center
Bronx, New York

Robert T. Brown, M.D.

Professor of Clinical Pediatrics
Professor of Clinical Obstetrics and Gynecology
The Ohio State University College of Medicine
Chief, Section of Adolescent Health
Children's Hospital
Columbus, Ohio

Volume 8/Number 3 October 1997
HANLEY & BELFUS, INC. Philadelphia

STATE OF THE ART REVIEWS

Publisher: HANLEY & BELFUS, INC.
Medical Publishers
210 South 13th Street
Philadelphia, PA 19107
(215) 546-7293
Fax (215) 790-9330
Internet: www.hanleyandbelfus.com

ADOLESCENT MEDICINE: State of the Art Reviews is indexed in the *Combined Cumulative Index to Pediatrics,* ISI/ISTP&B online database, Index to Scientific Book Contents, Biological Abstracts/RRM, and Current Contents (Clinical Medicine and Social & Behavioral Sciences).

ADOLESCENT MEDICINE: State of the Art Reviews ISSN 1041-3499
October 1997 Volume 8, Number 3 ISBN 1-56053-238-6

ADOLESCENT MEDICINE: State of the Art Reviews is published triannually (three times per year) by Hanley & Belfus, Inc., 210 South 13th Street, Philadelphia, Pennsylvania 19107.

POSTMASTER: Send address changes to ADOLESCENT MEDICINE: State of the Art Reviews, Hanley & Belfus, Inc., 210 South 13th Street, Philadelphia, PA 19107.

This issue is Volume 8, Number 3.

The Editor of this publication is Linda C. Belfus.

Adolescent Medicine: State of the Art Reviews

Official Journal of the
Section on Adolescent Health of the American Academy of Pediatrics

Adolescent Medicine: State of the Art Reviews

Official Journal of the
Section on Adolescent Health of the American Academy of Pediatrics

Instructions for Authors

Adolescent Medicine: State of the Art Reviews is the official journal of the Section on Adolescent Health of the American Academy of Pediatrics. Published three times a year, the journal features special topic-related issues with peer-reviewed articles by experts in particular fields. Although manuscripts are usually requested from specific authors based on the theme of each issue, others are welcome to query the Editors regarding their desire to write specific review articles or to guest edit an entire issue. Articles are peer-reviewed by 2 or more outside reviewers, experts in the particular field covered by the article, and manuscripts are closely edited as necessary.

Peer Review

Your manuscript will be reviewed by the guest editor, at least one of the editors-in-chief, and by members of the Editorial Board or Advisory Board, as appropriate. We ask your cooperation in accomplishing revisions expeditiously.

The Text

Three hard copies plus one diskette of the manuscript along with the original illustrations plus two photocopies of the illustrations should be sent to the guest editor. Unless otherwise indicated by the guest editor, the manuscript should be no longer than 20–25 double-spaced, typewritten pages, including references. Tables and figures are *not* included in the page count because they should be used wherever appropriate to enhance the text. The author's name and degrees, school and/or hospital appointments, mailing address, telephone number, and fax number *must* appear on the opening page.

Tables and Illustrations

Please consider the visual impact of your article. Tables and figures may be used to break up long blocks of text, and can be both informative and aesthetically pleasing.

Tables. Information given in tables may be commented upon but should not be repeated in the text. Each table should be numbered, given a brief descriptive title, typed on a separate sheet, and attached to the manuscript. Placement in the text should be indicated.

Illustrations. Avoid the use of fuzzy halftones or blurred photocopies of charts or graphs. Best results are obtained from original artwork or photographs in the form of glossy prints. Illustrations cannot be printed in color, but color prints may be submitted for conversion to black and white. One original plus two photocopies of each illustration, identified by marking lightly in pencil the figure number and author's name on the back, is sufficient. Do not mount illustrations with tape or glue or mark them with ball-point or felt-tipped pens. Legends should be typed on a separate sheet and attached to the manuscript. Placement in the text should be indicated.

References

References should be limited to 20 or 30 key sources unless an extensive review of the literature has been invited. References should be listed **alphabetically** rather than in order of occurrence, numbered for citation in the text, and typed double-spaced. Each reference should contain, in the order indicated, the author's last name and initials; the title of the article; the name of the periodical; and the volume, inclusive page numbers, and year. If a book is cited, give chapter author's name, chapter title, editor's name, title of book, place of publication, publisher, edition, and year. The *Index Medicus* abbreviations for journals should be used.

Borrowed Material

It is the author's responsibility to obtain letters of permission for borrowed material from both the publisher and the author of the original material. Copies of the letters granting permission should be forwarded to **Hanley & Belfus, Inc.** when they are received. Complete reference to original place of publication should be given in the legend to a borrowed figure or as a footnote to a borrowed table. Permission forms are available from the editor or publisher to expedite this process.

Proof

The first-named author of each article will receive page proof, unless otherwise specified, to be read carefully and returned to the publisher with only essential corrections. Please proofread your article carefully. Because of familiarity with the content, the author is the in the best position to identify substantive errors.

Complimentary Copies

Each contributor will receive a complimentary copy of the completed volume.

Contents

Contributors

Trina Menden Anglin, M.D., Ph.D.
Medical Officer, Office of Adolescent Health, Maternal and Child Health Bureau, Health Resources and Services Administration, Department of Health and Human Services, Rockville, Maryland

Carol Ford Arkin, Ph.D.
Postdoctoral Fellow, Department of Psychology, Columbus Children's Hospital, Columbus, Ohio

Jeff Q. Bostic, M.D., Ed.D.
Instructor in Psychiatry, Harvard Medical School, and Staff, Pediatric Psychopharmacology Clinic, Massachusetts General Hospital, Boston, Massachusetts

Karen J. Browner-Elhanan, M.D.
Postdoctoral Fellow, Department of Pediatrics, Division of Adolescent Medicine, Montefiore Medical Center and Albert Einstein College of Medicine, Bronx, New York

Mitchell D. Creinin, M.D.
Assistant Professor, Department of Obstetrics, Gynecology and Reproductive Sciences, University of Pittsburgh School of Medicine, and Magee-Women's Hospital, Pittsburgh, Pennsylvania

Nancy Neveloff Dubler, L.L.B.
Professor, Albert Einstein College of Medicine, and Director, Division of Bioethics, Department of Epidemiology and Social Medicine, Montefiore Medical Center, Bronx, New York

Jonathan M. Ellen, M.D.
Assistant Adjunct Professor of Pediatrics, Division of Adolescent Medicine, Department of Pediatrics, University of California San Francisco School of Medicine, San Francisco, California

Abigail English, J.D.
Director, Adolescent Health Care Project, National Center for Youth Law, Chapel Hill, North Carolina

J. Dennis Fortenberry, M.D., M.S.
Associate Professor of Pediatrics, Section of Adolescent Medicine, Department of Pediatrics, Indiana University School of Medicine, and Riley Hospital for Children, Indianapolis, Indiana

Jeffrey B. Gillman, Ph.D.
Department of Psychology, Columbus Children's Hospital, Columbus, Ohio

Melanie A. Gold, D.O.
Assistant Professor of Pediatrics, Department of Pediatrics, Children's Hospital of Pittsburgh, University of Pittsburgh School of Medicine, Pittsburgh, Pennsylvania

Bruce Greenstein, M.D.
Department of Plastic and Reconstructive Surgery, Albert Einstein College of Medicine, and Montefiore Medical Center, Bronx, New York

Jill E. Gurvey, M.P.H.
Division of Adolescent Medicine, Department of Pediatrics, University of California San Francisco School of Medicine, San Francisco, California

Geri D. Hewitt, M.D.
Clinical Assistant Professor of Obstetrics and Gynecology and Pediatrics, The Ohio State University College of Medicine, Ohio State University Medical Center, and Columbus Children's Hospital, Columbus, Ohio

Neal D. Hoffman, M.D.
Assistant Professor of Pediatrics, Albert Einstein College of Medicine, and Medical Director, Adolescent AIDS Program, Division of Adolescent Medicine, Montefiore Medical Center, Bronx, New York

Charles E. Irwin, Jr., M.D.
Professor of Pediatrics, Division of Adolescent Medicine, Department of Pediatrics, and National Adolescent Health Information Center, Institute of Health Policy, University of California San Francisco School of Medicine, San Francisco, California

Pamela J. Murray, M.D., M.H.P.
Associate Professor of Pediatrics, Department of Pediatrics, University of Pittsburgh School of Medicine; Director, Section of Adolescent Medicine, Children's Hospital of Pittsburgh, Pittsburgh, Pennsylvania

Marsha Maxine Quinn, J.D.
Division of Bioethics, Department of Epidemiology and Social Medicine, Montefiore Medical Center, Bronx, New York

Walter D. Rosenfeld, M.D.
Associate Professor of Clinical Pediatrics, College of Physicians and Surgeons of Columbia University; and Adolescent/Young Adult Center for Health, Morristown Memorial Hospital, Morristown, New Jersey

Paul Saenger, M.D.
Professor of Pediatrics, and Head, Division of Pediatric Endocrinology, Department of Pediatrics, Albert Einstein College of Medicine, and Montefiore Medical Center, Bronx, New York

S. Kenneth Schonberg, M.D.
Professor of Pediatrics, Albert Einstein College of Medicine, and Director, Division of Adolescent Medicine, Montefiore Medical Center, Bronx, New York

Victor C. Strasburger, M.D.
Professor of Pediatrics, and Chief, Division of Adolescent Medicine, University of New Mexico School of Medicine, Albuquerque, New Mexico

Berish Strauch, M.D.
Department of Plastic and Reconstructive Surgery, Albert Einstein College of Medicine, and Montefiore Medical Center, Bronx, New York

Gary A. Walco, Ph.D.
Associate Professor of Pediatrics, University of Medicine and Dentistry, New Jersey Medical School, Newark; Chief, Section of Pediatric Psychology, Hackensack University Medical Center, Hackensack, New Jersey

Esther H. Wender, MD.
Clinical Professor of Pediatrics, Albert Einstein College of Medicine, Bronx, New York

Charles J. Wibbelsman, M.D.
Associate Clinical Professor, Department of Pediatrics, University of California San Francisco; Chief, Teenage Clinic, Kaiser Permanente Medical Center, San Francisco, California

Timothy E. Wilens, M.D.
Associate Professor of Psychiatry, Harvard Medical School, and Staff, Pediatric Psychopharmacology Clinic, Massachusetts General Hospital, Boston, Massachusetts

Preface

Clinicians providing health care for adolescents encounter many problems and situations for which there are no clear-cut answers. These situations often are quite difficult to deal with practically, politically, and emotionally. This issue of **AM:STARs** explores several such *Controversies and Conundrums* and offers some cogent and stimulating discussions of the options available. From the pros and cons of medical abortion, to the use of growth hormone in normal short children, to discrimination in minority health care, we have not shied away from the controversial. We also present discussions of several conundrums in adolescent health that are infrequently addressed in the literature, including counseling the parents of rebellious teens, acculturation issues in immigrants, cosmetic plastic surgery, the diagnosis and treatment of ADHD, and many others. Authors were asked to clearly delineate conflicting opinions while feeling free to express their own points of view. Our intent as editors was and is to stimulate thought and discussion. Thank you to all the authors for sharing your views so eloquently. We hope our readers will find these penetrating glimpses into *Controversies and Conundrums* elucidating and, most importantly, clinically beneficial.

Susan M. Coupey, M.D.
Robert T. Brown, M.D.
GUEST EDITORS

1990–1997 Issues

1. **The At-Risk Adolescent**
   Edited by Victor C. Strasburger, M.D.
   Donald E. Greydanus, M.D.
2. **Adolescent Dermatology**
   Edited by Steven C. Shapiro, M.D.
   Victor C. Strasburger, M.D.
   Donald E. Greydanus, M.D.
3. **AIDS and Other Sexually Transmitted Diseases**
   Edited by Manuel Schydlower, M.D.
   Mary-Ann Shafer, M.D.
4. **Sports and the Adolescent**
   Edited by Paul G. Dyment, M.D.
5. **Parenting the Adolescent: Practitioner Concerns**
   Edited by George D. Comerci, M.D
   William A. Daniel, Jr., M.D.
6. **Acute and Chronic Medical Disorders**
   Edited by John W. Kulig, M.D., M.P.H.
7. **Psychosocial Issues in Adolescents**
   Edited by Robert T. Brown, M.D.
   Barbara A. Cromer, M.D.
8. **Adolescent Sexuality: Preventing Unhealthy Consequences**
   Edited by Susan M. Coupey, M.D.
   Lorraine V. Klerman, Dr.P.H.
9. **Adolescent Nutrition and Eating Disorders**
   Edited by Michael P. Nussbaum, M.D.
   Johanna Dwyer, D.Sc., R.D.
10. **Emergency Care of Adolescents**
    Edited by Stephen Ludwig, M.D.
    M. Susan Jay, M.D.
11. **Substance Abuse and Addictions**
    Edited by Manuel Schydlower, M.D.
    Peter Rogers, M.D.
12. **Adolescents and the Media**
    Edited by Victor C. Strasburger, M.D.
    George Comstock, Ph.D.
13. **Medical and Gynecologic Endocrinology**
    Edited by Joseph S. Sanfilippo, M.D.
    Jordan W. Finkelstein, M.D.
    Dennis M. Styne, M.D.
14. **Chronic and Disabling Disorders**
    Edited by Robert T. Brown, M.D.
    Susan M. Coupey, M.D.
15. **Adolescent Medicine and Health Care Delivery**
    Edited by Donald E. Greydanus, M.D.
16. **Viral Infections in Adolescents**
    Edited by Gary D. Overturf, M.D.
    Richard F. Jacobs, M.D.
17. **Violence and Injury Prevention**
    Edited by Katherine Kaufer Cristoffel, M.D., M.P.H.
    Carol W. Runyan, M.P.H., Ph.D.
18. **Gastrointestinal Disorders**
    Edited by Jeffrey S. Hymans, M.D.
19. **Male Reproductive Health**
    Edited by Paul G. Dyment, M.D.
20. **Health Care in Schools**
    Edited by Linda Juszczak, M.S., M.P.H., C.P.N.P., and Martin Fisher, M.D.
21. **Case Studies**
    Edited by John W. Kulig, M.D., M.P.H.
22. **Office-based Adolescent Health Care**
    Edited by Paula K. Braverman, M.D.
    Victor C. Strasburger, M.D.
23. **Gay and Lesbian Youth**
    Edited by Caitlin Ryan, M.S.W., A.S.C.W.
    Donna Futterman, M.D.
24. **Controversies and Conundrums**
    Edited by Susan M. Coupey, M.D.
    Robert T. Brown, M.D.

1998 Issues

25. **Rheumatologic Problems in Adolescents**
    Edited by George D. Comerci, M.D.
    Jane Schaller, M.D.
26. **Adolescent Psychiatric and Behavioral Disorders**
    Edited by Stanford B. Friedman, M.D.
    David De Maso, M.D.
27. **Office Orthopedics and Sports Medicine**
    Edited by Donald E. Greydanus, M.D., et al.

Subscriptions and single issues available from the publisher—Hanley & Belfus, Inc., Medical Publishers, 210 South 13th Street, Philadelphia, PA 19107, (215) 546-7293, fax (215) 790-9330.

Changing Health Care Environments and Adolescent Health Care: Legal and Policy Challenges

ABIGAIL ENGLISH, J.D.

Adolescent Health Care Project
National Center for Youth Law
Chapel Hill, North Carolina

Reprint requests to:
Abigail English, J.D.
Director, Adolescent Health Care Project
National Center for Youth Law
211 North Columbia Street
Chapel Hill, NC 27514

The pace of change in the health care arena in the United States has been accelerating at an astonishingly rapid rate. Adolescents, like other age groups, are affected by the changes. Even more than other groups, however, adolescents were already vulnerable to limitations on their access to necessary care. The risk exists that they will encounter some new obstacles in the current changing health care environments as well as the same ones that they have encountered all along. Overcoming this risk presents significant legal and policy challenges.

Two key areas of concern are the insurance status of adolescents and the shift to managed care. Dwindling coverage for children and adolescents in private employer-based health insurance plans and the explosion in the use of managed care by the public and private sectors have important implications for adolescents' access to health care. In the current climate, adolescents without adequate insurance are at greater risk than ever of limited access to care, and the extent to which managed care systems will meet adolescents' needs remains to be determined. Answers to several key questions will determine to a significant degree whether adolescents will receive the health care they need:

- Will adolescents have adequate health insurance?
- How will uninsured and underinsured adolescents receive care?
- Will managed care systems provide the benefits adolescents need most?
- Will confidentiality be protected?
- Will managed care plans and health care providers be accountable?

Many of these questions involve important legal and policy concerns, including many issues related to Medicaid, private insurance, and managed care organizations (MCOs).

WILL ADOLESCENTS HAVE ADEQUATE HEALTH INSURANCE?

A key feature of the changing health care environment is that having health insurance is an increasingly important element in access to care. People of any age who lack health insurance generally receive less health care.[14,27] While managed care systems hold out the promise of many potential benefits for adolescents and other age groups, adolescents who are not insured will not reap those benefits. Moreover, adolescents without any insurance or without insurance that covers the services they need increasingly will be unable to obtain those services without charge or at minimal cost, as they may have done in the past.

Insurance Status of Adolescents

Adolescents are uninsured at high rates and have been for some time. What is particularly worrisome, however, is that the situation is deteriorating. In 1988, 13.7% of adolescents ages 12–17 lacked health insurance,[18] and one in three adolescents living below the poverty level had no insurance.[19] Since then their insurance status has worsened. In 1992, 14.9% of adolescents ages 12–17 were uninsured. In 1993, 14% of adolescents ages 10–14, 19.9% of adolescents ages 15–18, and 25.2% of 19- to 21-year-olds were uninsured.9 The picture is even worse for certain groups of adolescents, such as those who are living below or just above the poverty level, who are living in the South, who are in fair or poor health, or who are members of racial or ethnic minority groups; all of these groups are uninsured at even higher rates than adolescents overall.[19]

Developments in Private Insurance and Medicaid

Over the past several years, health insurance coverage in private employer-based plans has decreased for children and adolescents. For example, from 1988–1992, adolescents ages 12–17 experienced a 7% decrease in employer-based insurance coverage.[18] From 1989–1995, the decrease in private insurance coverage resulted in a loss of private coverage for about 5 million children younger than 18.[26]

The Medicaid program has almost made up the difference in the loss of private insurance for younger children, but it has not done so for adolescents: even though Medicaid coverage of adolescents ages 12–17 increased by 27% from 1988–1992, the loss in private insurance was such that overall the percentage of adolescents who were uninsured increased by 9% during that period.[18] One reason Medicaid has done more to make up for losses in private coverage for younger children than for adolescents is that changes in Medicaid eligibility enacted by Congress in the late 1980s and early 1990s made it possible for some pregnant women and children to qualify based on their low income rather than their receipt of cash public assistance benefits, but these eligibility expansions did not fully include adolescents.[6]

While Congress required states to cover all pregnant women and children younger than 6 up to 133% of poverty, it only mandated that states phase in coverage of adolescents living below the poverty level 1 year at a time, and this phase-in will not be complete until 2002. States currently are required to cover only adolescents who are age 13 or younger.[6] Moreover, even the continued existence of the phase-in has been threatened. For example, when Congress voted in 1995 to convert the Medicaid program to a block grant (a measure vetoed by the President), it would have eliminated the mandatory phase-in; shortly thereafter, the National Governors Association proposed a restructuring of Medicaid that also would have made the phase-in optional rather than mandatory.[3,11]

Despite the uncertain status of the mandatory phase-in, some states have gone beyond the federal mandates and have used Medicaid options to expand coverage for adolescents. At least 23 states either have accelerated the phase-in, by increasing the age up to which poor adolescents can establish eligibility, or by raising the family income level up to which adolescents are covered, or both.[6,17]

Some programs at the state level provide health insurance for children who are not covered by private insurance plans or Medicaid.[17] These programs have followed a variety of models. Some are private ventures established and operated by private insurers, some involve state-private partnerships, and a few are state-funded programs.[13,27] Many of these programs are limited to ambulatory care services, and some limit coverage of benefits that are important to adolescents, such as mental health care.[27] Some programs cover only younger children and not adolescents.[27] In addition, numerous states have established initiatives that build on the existing Medicaid program, by picking up options in the Medicaid statute or obtaining a federal waiver to expand eligibility even further, using a combination of state and federal funding.[13,27]

Estimates of the number of children covered by the private and state-funded programs range from 40,000 children covered by private initiatives such as the Blue Cross "Caring for Children" programs to 250,000 children covered by the state-funded initiatives.[13,26] In any case, the number of adolescents receiving coverage through these programs is limited compared with the overall number who are uninsured. Important as these initiatives are, they are not a replacement for Medicaid coverage, both because of limitations in the benefits package they provide and because for the most part they do not function as entitlement programs; if funds run out during the year, there is no obligation to provide services.[27]

Federal Legislation to Expand Health Insurance Coverage for Children

A high level of attention to the problem of uninsured children resulted in a wave of proposals being introduced in Congress to expand health insurance coverage for uninsured children.[10] These proposals represented a range of different approaches, including a block grant to states to purchase private insurance policies for uninsured children and adolescents, creation of a new Medicare-type program for children, a voucher system that would enable families to purchase child-only private insurance policies, and an expansion of Medicaid to allow low-income families to buy into the program for their children.

On August 5, 1997, after extensive negotiation among Republicans and Democrats within Congress, and between Congress and the Administration, President Clinton signed legislation that includes a new federal child health expansion initiative.[2a] Proponents of the law suggest that it may enable states to cover as many as 5 million of the uninsured children in the United States.[2b]

The bill provides $24 billion to the states over five years, starting October 1, 1997. Funds will be distributed to states based on a formula that includes the state's percentage of low-income children, the state's percentage of uninsured low-income children, and the state's health care costs. States may spend the new funds to expand Medicaid, to create a new state child health program, or both. States must spend at least 90% of the funds to provide health insurance to children either through Medicaid or a new program. They may spend up to 10% of the funds for outreach, administrative costs, or direct purchase or provision of health services to children. States must match the new federal funds at a rate that is more favorable to the states than the regular Medicaid matching rate (i.e., 70% of the state's Medicaid rate, but no less than 15%). The favorable rate may be used for Medicaid expansion or in a new state child health insurance program.

States have flexibility in determining eligibility, benefits, and cost-sharing requirements. States may cover children and youth under age 19 in families with incomes under 200% of the federal poverty level (FPL) (or up to 50% higher than the Medicaid eligibility level in states that have raised Medicaid eligibility above 150% FPL). States must maintain their Medicaid eligibility levels that were in effect as of June 1, 1997. Only children who are not eligible for Medicaid may be covered under a new state child health program. The benefits for the Medicaid expansion are the benefits that are normally available to children under Medicaid. The benefits in a new state child health program must be the same as or "actuarially equivalent" to those in one of several "benchmark" plans (such as the plans available to federal or state employees or in large HMOs), none of which is as broad as Medicaid, or must be approved by DHHS. Cost-sharing in a new state child health program may not be imposed for well-baby care, well-child care, and immunizations. Cost-sharing for children in families with incomes below 150% FPL cannot be higher than allowed in Medicaid. Cost-sharing for children in families with higher incomes may be required on a sliding scale but cannot exceed 5% of family income.

The extent to which this new law is used to benefit adolescents will depend on decisions made at the state level, because the states have been given so much flexibility with respect to key issues. For example, states are permitted, but not required, to cover adolescents up through age 18; they are permitted, but not required, to establish a benefits package that includes the services adolescents need most; and they are permitted, but not required, to set cost-sharing requirements at levels that would enable adolescents to obtain confidential services on an independent basis. Whether these decisions are made favorably to adolescents will depend on the work of advocates, health care providers, and state officials over the coming months and years. Because federal funds become available beginning October 1, 1997, many of these decisions, at least initially, will be made very quickly.

HOW WILL UNINSURED AND UNDERINSURED ADOLESCENTS RECEIVE CARE?

Adolescents who have no health insurance, whose coverage is inadequate, or who cannot access their families' coverage for services they need on a confidential basis have been able to obtain care at a variety of sites and from a range of providers who provide services without charge or on a sliding scale.[6] These sites include teen clinics, hospital-based adolescent medicine departments, community-based public health clinics, school-based and school-linked clinics, and family planning sites. The providers, sometimes referred to as essential community providers, have been able to provide uncompensated or low-cost care to uninsured and underinsured adolescents. However, the sources of funds for these programs, usually categorical grants for specific services such as family planning or public health services, are increasingly scarce and the competition for them has intensified.[6] Thus, financial survival for such providers depends more on third-party reimbursement and on the ability to obtain managed care contracts and to join the provider networks of managed care organizations.[4] The funds received through these mechanisms, however, do not enable the providers to offer free care to adolescents who are not insured or enrolled in managed care. As a result, it will become more difficult for adolescents without adequate insurance to find free or low-cost care.

WILL MANAGED CARE SYSTEMS PROVIDE THE BENEFITS ADOLESCENTS NEED MOST?

Not only are too few adolescents currently insured, but even those who have health insurance may lack coverage for essential services. Even when services are nominally covered in the Medicaid or private managed care plan in which the adolescent is enrolled, it may be difficult for an adolescent to access the services, because of limitations on the providers an enrolled adolescent may use, restrictive medical necessity criteria, and prior authorization or utilization review procedures.

Scope of Benefits in Medicaid and Private Plans

Medicaid covers a broad range of medically necessary services; some are mandatory for all states, and others may be offered at the state's option. For Medicaid-eligible children and adolescents through age 20, the benefits package is a comprehensive one that includes many of the physical, mental, and developmental health services they need. Indeed, since 1989, as a result of the Early and Periodic Screening, Diagnosis, and Treatment (EPSDT) requirements of the Medicaid statute, states must cover any mandatory or optional federal Medicaid service that is medically necessary to meet the needs of eligible children and adolescents.[2] This means that, officially at least, adolescents who are eligible for Medicaid should be able to obtain a full range of preventive services, reproductive health care other than abortion, mental and behavioral health services, and care for chronic illness or disability. However, because implementation has lagged behind program requirements, not all Medicaid-eligible adolescents are receiving the comprehensive care to which they are entitled.

The comprehensive Medicaid benefits package should be available to eligible adolescents whether they are enrolled in Medicaid on the traditional fee-for-service basis or in a Medicaid managed care plan. However, variations on the theme do occur. For example, in the contracts between Medicaid agencies and managed care organizations, the provisions specifying the covered services vary widely in terms of the degree to which services important to adolescents are specifically spelled out.[6] In addition, some services (e.g., for behavioral health or treatment of the human immunodeficiency virus) may be "carved out" of the standard Medicaid managed care plan and offered separately through a different capitated plan or on a fee-for-service basis.[6] In light of the varied arrangements states have established for making the full range of Medicaid benefits available to eligible adolescents, there is a significant risk that, without sufficient coordination, some benefits will be missed by some adolescents.

Private health insurance plans, including managed care plans, vary dramatically in the scope of benefits they cover. These variations occur as the result of decisions made both by the purchasers of health insurance coverage (e.g., employers) and by the plans themselves (e.g., pricing structures for inclusion of different services). Many of the variations are significant for adolescents. For example, recent studies document that the range of reproductive health services covered by managed care plans differs significantly among the various models of managed care.[8] Reports by providers suggest that some private insurers will cover chlamydia screening only for symptomatic adolescents and that others are not covering hepatitis B and other immunizations for teens.[6]

A number of states have enacted laws governing health maintenance organizations (HMOs) or other managed care organizations that mandate inclusion of certain benefits.

Although the scope of these mandates varies widely, some states have required coverage for certain preventive services and others that are important to adolescents.[6]

Access to Adolescent-Focused Providers

Even when a Medicaid or private managed care plan covers a comprehensive benefits package, adolescents' access to the services may depend on many other factors. One key consideration is whether adolescent-focused or adolescent-friendly providers—who have the training, experience, and interest in caring for this age group—are included in a managed care plan's network of providers. If they are included, an additional issue is whether adolescents must overcome significant hurdles to use them. Again, significant variations characterize current practice.

Managed care plans have no consistent or predictable policies about whether health care professionals with expertise in adolescent medicine are included in plan networks or, if they are included, whether they are classified as primary care providers, specialists, or both. Such providers serve important functions in each capacity, but many plans either require them to choose one classification or the plan makes the classification for them. Few legal requirements address this issue. In the model contracts between state Medicaid agencies and managed care organizations, for example, few states explicitly require MCOs to include adolescent medicine providers in their networks, and only a few mandate that MCOs consult or enter into subcontracts with school-based health centers.[6] However, even in some states where school-based centers are included in managed care provider networks, adolescents may need to obtain a referral from their primary care provider/gatekeeper to be able to use the centers' services.[6]

Medical Necessity, Prior Authorization, and Utilization Review

Even assuming that managed care plans cover an appropriate and comprehensive range of benefits and that adolescent-focused providers are included in plan networks, adolescents nevertheless may encounter other barriers in their efforts to obtain needed services. Limitations on the availability of services in specific circumstances may take the form of restrictive definitions of medical necessity or burdensome prior authorization or utilization review procedures.

The Medicaid program's operative definition of medical necessity for children and adolescents through age 20 is contained in the EPSDT provision of the Medicaid statute. It is one of the broadest definitions of medical necessity used in any public or private health insurance plan, requiring coverage of screening, preventive, diagnostic, and treatment services that are necessary to address physical, mental, and developmental problems.[2] In contrast, some managed care plans use more restrictive medical necessity definitions, permitting coverage only for services necessary to treat an illness or injury, for example.[7] Although by federal statute the EPSDT standard must be applied for all Medicaid-eligible children and adolescents through age 20, Medicaid managed care contracts do not always make this clear. Only a few state contracts include explicit provisions to this effect, and some MCOs with contracts to serve the Medicaid population are continuing to use their more restrictive definitions.[6,7]

Numerous reports from health care providers who serve adolescents suggest that prior authorization procedures sometimes function as obstacles to the provision of appropriate services.[6] In particular, mental health services and services needed to address eating disorders have been cited as ones that often trigger denials by prior authorization personnel. One reason may be that the MCO's staff members who are responsible for prior authorization are rarely trained in the specific health care needs of adolescents.

WILL CONFIDENTIALITY BE PROTECTED?

One specific need that characterizes the adolescent age group is the desire for protection of confidentiality in health care.[24] This is both an expression of normal adolescent development and a reflection of the sensitivity of the health care concerns for which adolescents are seeking care. Effective protection of confidentiality depends on the operation of several factors. First, for confidentiality to be fully protected, adolescents must be able to obtain care based on their own consent. Second, financial arrangements must be in place that do not require adolescents to assume unrealistic cost-sharing burdens. Finally, procedures designed to provide effective protection for confidentiality must be implemented by MCOs.

Every state has at least some laws that authorize minors to consent to care based either on their status (e.g., as emancipated or mature minors) or on the services they seek (e.g., contraceptive services, care for sexually transmitted diseases, or substance abuse treatment).[5] These laws are not universally known or well understood by many insurers, MCOs, and even some health care providers. In particular, to the extent that managed care provider networks are composed primarily of those who do not customarily serve adolescents, lack of familiarity with the consent laws regarding minors creates obstacles to confidentiality. Similarly, if MCOs do not recognize the right of minors to consent to their own care in specific circumstances, they will be unable to obtain confidential care on an independent basis.

A major barrier for adolescents trying to obtain confidential health care is the necessity for involving third parties, including parents, in the payment for services. Few, if any, insurers will process a dependent's claim without a signature from the insured, usually a parent. However, adolescents seeking sensitive services—for a sexually transmitted disease or contraception—may be unwilling to involve their parents. Even if, as in many prepaid health plans, a claim form requiring a parent's signature does not need to be filed, the copayments that must be made at the time of service for office visits, laboratory work, or prescription drugs may be high enough to prevent adolescents from using the services independently.[4] In addition, statements from the insurance company or MCO may subsequently be sent to families.

Finally, protecting the confidentiality of health care information—both oral communications and written records—is a challenge for any age group of patients, but particularly for adolescents. For managed care organizations to succeed in doing so, they must develop and implement procedures that take account of the specific needs of this age group. Some HMOs, for example, that have established teen clinics also have established special protections for the confidentiality of records that contain information about sensitive services received by adolescent patients in those clinics.[4]

Adolescents' perceptions of the degree of confidentiality are nearly as important as the actual degree of protection that is in place. On the one hand, even a perception on the part of adolescents that confidentiality is not protected may be enough to prompt them to seek care at other sites.[4] Therefore, it is important for MCOs and their providers to make the confidentiality protections known to adolescents. On the other hand, confidentiality protection cannot be absolute. For instance, disclosure is required when an adolescent is suicidal or for the purpose of mandatory child abuse reporting—and adolescents should not be misled about the scope of confidentiality protection they can expect.[25]

WILL MANAGED CARE PLANS BE ACCOUNTABLE?

Whatever the standards and procedures for establishing the benefits package, authorizing access to providers and services, or protecting confidentiality, it is essential that managed care plans be held accountable for adhering to them and for meeting their contractual obligations. Professional guidelines for the delivery of appropriate services to the adolescent population, particularly preventive services, have been developed.[23] There is broad consensus among these guidelines concerning the appropriate content of services.[23] A few of the elements contained in the guidelines also have been incorporated into performance measures currently in use in the managed care arena, but many have not. In addition, some existing legal provisions would require reporting of data by MCOs that would help to hold them accountable, but these provisions have not been implemented consistently.

Adolescent-oriented Performance Measures

The numerous guidelines for adolescent health services that have been endorsed by a broad spectrum of professional groups are based to a significant degree on data documenting the burden of suffering associated with adolescent risk behaviors as well as expert opinion concerning how to reduce these behavioral risks.[12] No comprehensive set of indicators based on these guidelines has yet been adopted as a yardstick for measuring the performance of managed care plans. From the perspective of some entities, such as MCOs or state Medicaid agencies, the performance measures used to hold managed care plans accountable should be based on the efficacy and cost-effectiveness of the indicators that are used. While such evidence is not readily available for the full range of professionally recommended adolescent health services, there are specific services that meet these criteria,[24] including certain immunizations, screening for *Chlamydia trachomatis* and cervical cancer, and contraceptive services.

One of the leading sets of indicators that is used to evaluate the performance of managed care plans is the Health Plan Employer Data and Information Set (HEDIS) measures developed by the National Committee for Quality Assurance. HEDIS was originally developed for the private arena, but a version for Medicaid managed care plans was later issued.[16] The most recent version, HEDIS 3.0, is designed for use with both private and Medicaid managed care plans.[15] A few adolescent-specific indicators were included, for the first time, in Medicaid HEDIS, and a few more were added in HEDIS 3.0. The adolescent-specific indicators in HEDIS 3.0 include hepatitis B, varicella, and a second dose of measles, mumps, rubella vaccinations; annual comprehensive well-care visits; cervical cancer screening; substance use counseling; and chlamydia screening (a measure that is still in the testing phase).[15]

In addition to any obligation Medicaid managed care plans may have to comply with HEDIS requirements, they also are usually required to adhere to the mandates of the Medicaid statute, particularly because many of the contracts between state Medicaid agencies and managed care plans explicitly incorporate those requirements by reference. These mandates include reporting requirements that would promote the accountability of managed care plans. Medicaid-eligible adolescents through age 20 are entitled to the full range of services represented by the EPSDT benefit, including annual comprehensive health exams.[2] States are required to submit data annually to the Health Care Financing Administration (HCFA) documenting the extent of compliance with EPSDT requirements.[1] These requirements are as relevant for adolescents enrolled in Medicaid managed care plans as for those whose care is reimbursed on a fee-for-service basis.

Implementation of Existing Requirements

While some progress has been made toward the inclusion of adolescent-specific measures in some of the efforts to ensure accountability on the part of managed care plans, these efforts are still in a preliminary phase. Moreover, the actual implementation of requirements such as those included in HEDIS 3.0, as well as the statutory requirements applicable to the Medicaid program, has been uneven. Few states thus far have incorporated HEDIS indicators into their Medicaid managed care contracts, and neither HCFA nor state Medicaid agencies have adopted a vigorous stance toward enforcement of the statutory reporting requirements applicable to the provision of EPSDT services by managed care plans. A few states, however, have undertaken some innovations on their initiative. For example, Massachusetts has made adherence to EPSDT screening requirements a performance measure for its Medicaid HMOs and is moving toward enforcement of a requirement for annual comprehensive health assessments for adolescents.[6]

CONCLUSION

Although the visibility of adolescent health issues has increased over the past decade through the efforts of numerous organizations, agencies, and individuals, adolescents remain vulnerable to limitations on access to health care. In the current changing health care environment, the way in which we meet the legal and policies challenges with respect to two issues—the insurance status of adolescents and the shift to managed care—will affect adolescents' access to health care to a significant degree. Without insurance coverage, adolescents will receive no benefits from managed care and increasingly may encounter obstacles to obtaining free or low-cost care apart from insurance coverage. For adolescents who are insured and enrolled in managed care plans, the benefits they derive will depend on the extent to which managed care organizations are willing to learn about the needs of this age group and adapt their services and procedures to meet the needs.

References

1. 42 U.S.C. § 1396a(a)(43).
2. 42 U.S.C. § 1396d(r).

2a. Balanced Budget Act of 1997, Pub. L. No. 105–33, 111 Stat. 251 (1997).

2b. Clinton HR: New era in health coverage for children. The News and Observer, Aug. 6, 1997, p 15A.

3. Balanced Budget Act of 1995, H.R. 2491, 104th Cong. 2nd Sess., passed Nov. 20, 1995; and Congressional Record, H12557–H12582, Nov. 15, 1995 (containing the Medicaid provisions of H.R. 2491).
4. English A, Kapphahn C, Perkins J, Wibbelsman CJ: Meeting the health care needs of adolescents in managed care: A position paper of the Society for Adolescent Medicine. J Adolesc Health (in press).
5. English A, Matthews M, Extavour K, et al: State Minor Consent Statutes: A Summary. Cincinnati, OH, Center for Continuing Education in Adolescent Health, 1995.
6. English A, Perkins J, Teare C, et al: Adolescent Health Care in Transition: Medicaid, Managed Care, and Health Care Reform. San Francisco, National Center for Youth Law (in press).
7. Fox HB, McManus MA: Impacts of State Medicaid Demonstration Waiver Programs on Children—Results from Hawaii, Oregon, Rhode Island, and Tennessee. Washington, D.C., Fox Health Policy Consultants, 1996.
8. Gold RB, Richards C: Improving the Fit: Reproductive Health Services in Managed Care. New York, Alan Guttmacher Institute, 1996.
9. Hughes D: Health Insurance Trends Among Children: 1988 and 1993: Unpublished Tabulations from the Current Population Survey. San Francisco, Institute for Health Policy Studies, 1996.
10. Johnson K, DeGraw C, Sonosky C, et al: Children's Health Insurance: A Comparison of Major Federal Legislation. Washington, D.C., George Washington University Center for Health Policy Research, 1997.
11. King MP, Christian SM: Medicaid Survival Kit. Denver, National Conference of State Legislatures, November 1996.
12. Klein J, Elster A, Hedberg V, et al: Implications for public health surveillance and managed care quality improvement measuring clinical preventive services delivery for adolescents [unpublished manuscript].
13. Mann C, Ross DC, Cox L: The Medicaid Program Has Been the Program of Choice for Most States That Have Expanded Coverage for Uninsured Children. Washington, D.C., Center on Budget and Policy Priorities, 1997.

14. Monheit AC, Cunningham PJ: Children without health insurance. The Future of Children 2(2):154, Winter 1992, p 154.
15. National Committee for Quality Assurance: HEDIS 3.0. Washington, DC., NCQA, 1997.
16. National Committee for Quality Assurance: Medicaid HEDIS: An Adaptation of NCQA's Health Plan Employer Data and Information Set 2.0/2.5. Washington, D.C., NCQA, 1995.
17. National Governors' Association: New State Efforts to Provide Health Care Coverage for Uninsured Children—Spring 1997. Stateline, April 22, 1997.
18. Newacheck PW, Hughes D, Cisternas M: Children and health insurance: An overview of recent trends. Health Affairs 14:244–254, 1995.
19. Newacheck PW, McManus MA, Gephart J: Health insurance coverage of adolescents: A current profile and assessment of trends. Pediatrics 90:589–596, 1992.
20. Perkins J: Financing issues in Medicaid managed care. In Langill D, Dubois SK, Martin K, et al (eds): Medicaid Managed Care: An Advocate's Guide for Protecting Children. Washington, D.C., National Association of Child Advocates, 1996, pp 5-1–5-32.
21. Rivera L: Ensuring access to services in Medicaid managed care. In Langill D, Dubois SK, Martin K, et al (eds): Medicaid Managed Care: An Advocate's Guide for Protecting Children. Washington, D.C., National Association of Child Advocates, 1996. pp 4-1–4-52.
22. Rivera L: Ensuring quality in Medicaid managed care. In Langill D, Dubois SK, Martin K, et al (eds): Medicaid Managed Care: An Advocate's Guide for Protecting Children. Washington, D.C., National Association of Child Advocates, 1996, pp 6-1–6-30.
23. Rosen DS, Elster A, Hedberg V, Paperny D: Clinical preventive services for adolescents: Position paper of the Society for Adolescent Medicine. J Adolesc Health (in press).
24. Santelli J, Vernon M, Lowry R, et al: A Working Paper on School and Adolescent Health Services [draft]. Atlanta, Centers for Disease Control and Prevention, 1997.
25. Sigman G, Silber T, English A, Gans J: Confidential health care for adolescents: Position paper of the Society for Adolescent Medicine. J Adolesc Health (in press).
26. U.S. General Accounting Office: Employment-Based Health Insurance: Costs Increase and Family Coverage Decreases. Washington, D.C., GAO, 1997, publication HEHS-97-35.
27. U.S. General Accounting Office: Health Insurance for Children: State and Private Programs Create New Strategies to Insure Children. Washington, D.C., GAO, 1996, publication HEHS-96-35.

Discrimination in Minority Health Care

JONATHAN M. ELLEN, M.D.
JILL E. GURVEY, M.P.H.
CHARLES E. IRWIN, JR., M.D.

Division of Adolescent Medicine
Department of Pediatrics
and
National Adolescent Health Information Center
Department of Pediatrics and Institute for Health Policy
School of Medicine
University of California, San Francisco
San Francisco, California

Reprint requests to:
Jonathan M. Ellen, M.D.
1350 7th Avenue, Room 235
San Francisco, CA 94143-0848

The authors were supported in part by the Maternal and Child Health Bureau (grants MCJ000978A and MCJ063A80), Rockville, Maryland, and the National Institute of Allergy and Infectious Diseases (grant AI3499), Bethesda, Maryland.

Since 1990, the population of adolescents 10 to 19 years old has grown steadily. A greater proportion of this growth has occurred among racial/ethnic minorities.[72] Although adolescence is characterized by relatively good health, racial/ethnic minority adolescents are less healthy than white, non-Hispanic adolescents. Minority youth report a lower general health status (Table 1); experience a higher prevalence of many infectious diseases, including sexually transmitted diseases (STDs) and human immunodeficiency virus (HIV); and are more likely to die from homicide and HIV infection (Table 2). Although racial/ethnic differences in individual health-compromising behaviors account, in part, for differing morbidity and mortality rates,[52,63] failures of the traditional health care system to address the unique needs of minority youth may contribute to their poorer health status.

Data suggest that racial/ethnic minority youth may be less likely to receive quality primary care than white, non-Hispanic youth.[28,34,47] This discrimination in health care may be attributable to the demonstrable differences in factors associated with minority race/ethnicity, including differing cultural views on health, lower socioeconomic position, and geographic segregation.[39] This chapter explores how these factors affect minority adolescents' health status. The first half of this chapter outlines many of the racial/ethnic differences in culture, neighborhoods, and socioeconomic positions and describes the direct link between the latter two factors and health status. The second half of the chapter describes how these factors may interfere with health care delivery to minority adolescents.

TABLE 1. Health Status of United States Adolescents by Race, 1988

Health Status	White (%)	Black (%)	Hispanic (%)	All Adolescents (%)
Excellent or very good	83	61	74	78
Good, fair, or poor	17	39	26	22

Adapted from Lieu TA, Newacheck PW, McManus MA: Race, ethnicity, and access to ambulatory care among US adolescents. Am J Public Health 83:960–965, 1993, with permission.

DEMOGRAPHICS

The number of adolescents in the United States is growing even though the proportion of adolescents in the general population has remained static. In 1995 there were nearly 37 million adolescents, 14.1% of the United States population.[72] This figure increased by more than 2 million from 1990 to 1995. In addition, the racial/ethnic minorities are overrepresented among adolescents compared with the general population. For example, 12% of the U.S. population is black, but 15% of adolescents are black. Latinos, Asian/Pacific Islanders, and Native Americans constitute approximately 9.8%, 3.4%, and 0.007%, respectively, of the overall United States population but comprise 12%, 4%, and 1% of adolescents.[72]

SOCIOECONOMIC POSITION

Low household income, low educational attainment, and nonprofessional occupational status are socioeconomic characteristics associated with minority race/ethnicity, and these factors are associated with worse health[1,34,41,53,63,81] and less access to health insurance.[28,47] In addition, at all levels of socioeconomic position, racial/ethnic minorities generally have poorer health than whites.[24,31,41,48,63,81]

TABLE 2. Seven Leading Causes of Death among 15- to 24-Year-Olds in the United States, by Race and Sex, 1994

White		Black		Hispanic*
Male	Female	Male	Female	
Accidents†	Accidents†	Homicide	Homicide	Homicide
Suicide	Homicide	Accidents†	Accidents†	Accidents†
Homicide	Malignant neoplasm	Suicide	HIV	Suicide
Malignant neoplasm	Suicide	HIV	Heart disease	Malignant neoplasm
Heart disease	Heart disease	Heart disease	Malignant neoplasm	Heart disease
HIV	Congenital anomalies	Malignant neoplasm	Suicide	HIV
Congenital anomalies	Pneumonia and influenza	Chronic obstructive pulmonary disease	Complications of pregnancy and childbirth	Congenital anomalies

Adapted from Singh GK, Kochanek KD, MacDorman MF: Advance report of final mortality statistics, 1994. Monthly vital statistics report; 45(3), suppl. Hyattsville, MD, National Center for Health Statistics, 1996.
* Not available by sex.
† Accidents include motor vehicle accidents.

The degree to which parental education or occupation influences adolescents' health is largely unknown.[31] However, highly educated parents or parents engaged in professional occupations (i.e., parents with higher socioeconomic status) may be more able to provide social support and to create a healthier environment for their adolescent.[1] These factors could improve the health of adolescents.

Income and Poverty Status

The 1994 median family incomes for blacks and Latinos were $21,027 and $23,421, respectively, compared with $34,028 for whites.[71] During the same year, 44% of black, 42% of Latino, and 17% of white children younger than 18 lived at or below the poverty line. Asians/Pacific Islanders had a median income of $40,482, considerably higher than any other racial/ethnic group; however, this figure may be artificially high due to those families having a larger number of workers per household.[48] It also masks the differences in income between the different Asian subgroups; for example, the median income of Vietnamese and other Southeast Asians in the United States is about half of that of the overall Asian/Pacific Islander population.[48]

Educational Attainment

There are also racial/ethnic differences in the educational attainment of adults.[74] In 1995, 84.1% of Asian/Pacific Islanders, 83% of whites, 73.8% of blacks, and 53.4% of Latinos completed high school. College degrees and more advanced degrees were attained by whites at almost twice the rate of blacks (24% vs. 13%). Only 9.3% of Latinos attained college and more advanced degrees. Nearly 40% of Asian/Pacific Islanders completed college.

Occupational Status

There are substantial racial/ethnic differences in occupational status. Whites are overrepresented among the traditionally upper-class career positions compared with their number in the general population.[75] These occupations are associated with better health status.[38] Of employed adults 25–64 years old who occupy managerial or professional positions, 7.5% are black and 88% are white. In addition, blacks in professional positions earn a salary that is 75% of the salary of whites in the same job category. Within working-class jobs, blacks earn 63% of the salary of whites.

Family Structure

Blacks are more likely to reside in single-parent households than whites.[45] In 1995, 64% of black children and 25% of white children younger than 18 came from single-parent households.[74] Independent of poverty status, adolescents residing in single-parent households are more likely to report being in poor health.[41]

Interaction of Race/Ethnicity and Socioeconomic Position

Lower socioeconomic position and minority race/ethnicity have interactive effects on health. Poor minority adolescents are more likely to be unhealthy than poor white youth. According to data from the 1980 and 1984 National Health Interview Surveys (NHIS), the highest proportion of children who were rated to be in poor or fair health were black children living in poverty.[41] In studies of adult mortality, blacks have higher mortality rates than whites at each level of income and education.[53,67] Latinos' mortality rates and overall health status more closely resemble those of whites despite the fact that Latinos' poverty and education levels are similar to those of blacks. The apparent lack of association between socioeconomic factors and health among Latinos has been referred to as an "epidemiologic paradox."[37] One possible explanation for this phenomenon is that Latinos who have recently immigrated are buffered from the effects of their lower socioeconomic position by their low levels of acculturation.[36] With increasing assimilation into American culture, i.e., increasing acculturation, the health status of Latinos begins to approach that of blacks.

Health Insurance

Racial/ethnic minority adolescents are less likely to have health insurance than white adolescents. According to estimates from the 1988 NHIS, 86% of adolescents have some type of health insurance. About 16% of black adolescents, 28% of Latino adolescents, and 11% of white adolescents were uninsured.[34] In a study conducted by the Robert Wood Johnson Foundation, researchers found that among children younger than 18, the likelihood of having health insurance was decreased if the child was poor (< 100% federal poverty level), near-poor (100–150% federal poverty level), or belonged to a racial/ethnic minority.[82]

NEIGHBORHOODS

The health of minority youths is at greater risk because of the types of neighborhoods in which they reside. From the 1930s to the 1970s, the growth of suburban populations was massive.[51] However, blacks and other minority groups remained in urban centers, where the living standards are lower.[39] Data from 1984 show that 33% of adolescents living in urban areas but only 19% of those living in nonurban areas belonged to a minority group.[72]

Inner-city neighborhoods are often characterized by crowded conditions, which increase the risk of the spread of infectious diseases such as tuberculosis.[48] Children who live in run-down buildings typical of inner-city housing are more likely to have been exposed to lead-based paint, which may contribute to cognitive impairments.[46] The incidence of gun-related violence is also higher in urban areas.[10,61] Environmentally hazardous industrial operations are often located near poor or working-class neighborhoods.[20] Living near such industry has been associated with an increased risk of respiratory problems and possibly breast cancer.[21] Poor urban neighborhoods also have an excess of tobacco and alcohol advertisements.[4,22,42,62,77,79] Finally, these neighborhoods lack quality primary care, which may indirectly influence the health of adolescents.[30,82]

CULTURAL VIEWS ON HEALTH

Minority youth come from a variety of cultural backgrounds. Cultural background influences health beliefs and health values.[12,14,29,50,65] While there is great diversity in the health beliefs of the members of different racial/ethnic minorities in America, a few major themes emerge that distinguish the cultural beliefs of blacks, Latinos, and Asian Americans from those of the predominantly white health care system.[49] These themes include their definitions of disease and illness,[29,55,59,70] treatment and prevention practices,[14,40,58,66] the importance of family,[15,50,57,69] and the relationship between patient and physician.[12,13,54,65] Below we summarize how these belief systems are expressed in different cultures. Due to the lack of available data, this discussion does not cover the extensive variation in culture within racial/ethnic groups. Furthermore, there may be more commonalities in health beliefs among adolescents from different races/ethnicities but similar socioeconomic position than there are among their parents and families.

Definitions of Illness

The traditional health care system focuses on the diagnoses and treatment of diseases. Diseases are defined as abnormalities in the physiology and function of body organs and systems.[29] Lay people, especially those from non-Western cultures, focus more on illnesses. Ilness is the experience of undesirable changes in social functioning and state of being.[29] While traditional medicine explains diseases in terms of biology, non-western cultures' explanations for illnesses often involve the interplay between biology and spiritual or supernatural forces. Chinese Americans view health as the harmonious interplay among the body, the spirit or soul, and nature.[59] Illnesses represent an imbalance in these relationships, and treatments are directed at restoring this balance.[50] Not surprisingly, Chinese Americans favor more holistic treatment methods, which include herbal remedies and acupuncture.[50] In addition, some Asian cultures place a heavy emphasis on stoicism and the inevitability of illness.[40,70]

Latinos' views on health and illness stem from their strong religious backgrounds. Many Latinos believe that health is a "gift from God" and that illnesses are a form of punishment from God or invasions of evil spirits.[15,58] For example, a pain in the stomach or loss of appetite may be the symptoms of *susto* (Fright), and it is thought to be a result of an invasion of outside spirits or the soul leaving the body and needing to be coaxed back.[58] Mexican Americans rely on non-Western forms of "folk" medicine, such as *curanderismo*, which uses a religious and social model of health rather than a biomedical model.[15] Treatments often include prayer or the work of a religious healer to drive away evil.[65] Latinos also believe that some illnesses are a result of an imbalance in the body between hot and cold. Arthritis is a "cold" ailment, and ulcers and rashes are "hot" ailments.[65] Treatment of these ailments is directed at restoring this balance. Hot foods are prescribed when "cold" illnesses occur and vice versa.

Finally, blacks also have a history of believing in the supernatural and practicing folk medicine.[27,66] However, it is unclear to what extent beliefs in nontraditional methods of healing stem from a cultural epistemology rooted in African or Caribbean culture or represent a response to their experience with racism in the health care system.[27,69]

Role of the Family

There is a difference between how traditional medicine and non-Western cultures recognize the importance of family. Traditional health care providers see the family as peripheral to the treatment of patients. Most non-Western cultures view the family as integral to health-related decision-making and treatment. As such, traditional medicine often overlooks this necessary element of a successful treatment plan.

The concept of the individual is nonexistent in Asian cultures; in Chinese, there is no equivalent word for *self*.[49] Individuality is looked down upon in favor of the "collective" interest, which is usually that of the extended family or larger community. In Asian cultures, the family's well-being is often placed before the individual. In a study of terminally ill cancer patients, Korean American participants reported that it is the family and not the patient who should hear the diagnosis of the disease and decide whether or not to continue life support.[5] Furthermore, Asian families are patriarchal.[69] Men make all the important decisions regarding medical treatments. As such, it would be inappropriate to ask a woman to make a medical decision independent of a husband or father.[50]

The family is the central entity in Latino culture as well. *Familismo* (familism) describes the Mexican American concept of strong kin relationships.[23] As in Asian culture, health remedies are often provided by family members. Research has shown that *familismo* affects health-seeking behaviors.[23,54,57] Latino culture is also patriarchal. One study found that among Puerto Rican women, issues of male dominance and modesty influenced how they used preventive gynecologic services; those who were more modest and reported higher male dominance were less likely to get preventive gynecologic care.[54]

The extended family also is a very important aspect of black culture.[27,69] Often, family members including aunts, cousins, and grandparents play instrumental roles in raising children and providing economic, social, and emotional support. In contrast to other cultures, gender roles are more fluid in African American families, resulting in a less patriarchal family structure.[69] Mothers, grandmothers, or other female family members may be the primary decision-makers regarding health. This may be a result of the increased proportion of black households in the United States that are headed by women.

Interaction with the Health Care System

Racial/ethnic differences in culture may affect provider-patient communication and act as barriers to effective interactions with the health care system.[33,50,57,65] Traditional health care stresses patient autonomy.[5] This is often at odds with the non-Western belief that physicians are the authority. Latino patients expect the provider to identify "what's wrong" rather than to ask questions concerning symptoms. The concept of *patrón-peón* is the idea that all relationships have hierarchies. Latinos assume their doctor is in a position of authority over them and may be put off if the physician does not act accordingly.[57,65] However, directness and bluntness are considered to be rude and disrespectful and to violate the concept of *respeto*.[65]

Many blacks have an overall mistrust of the health care system,[17] which may affect their use of and interaction with the health care system.[33] This mistrust is likely rooted in the history of institutional racism within health care that dates back to the mid 1800s.[25,60] During that time, medical researchers subjected black slaves to inhumane conditions "in the name of science."[25] A more recent instance of such racism was the infamous federally guided Tuskeegee syphilis study, which began in 1932 and continued for more than 40 years.[7] In this study, researchers secretly and deliberately withheld treatment (including penicillin when it became available) from an all-black sample of men to document "the natural history of the disease." Many of the current structural barriers to accessible and available health care are perceived by blacks as a continuation of racism within traditional health care.

HEALTH CARE DELIVERY AND UTILIZATION

Evidence suggests that racial/ethnic minority youth may have a greater need for quality primary care because they are more likely than white, non-Hispanic youth to reside in impoverished, isolated, hazardous neighborhoods and to come from socioeconomically disadvantaged households. The same factors coupled with differences in beliefs about health, illness, and the health care system may limit the ability of the traditional health care system to respond to these needs. This section outlines where such barriers may exist using the Society of Adolescent Medicine's definition of quality primary care as a framework. According to the society, effective health care delivery should have the following features: availability and affordability, confidentiality, quality, cultural competency, and coordination and comprehensiveness.[28]

Availability and Affordability

Primary health care may be less available to minority adolescents. Inner-city neighborhoods are often cut off geographically from health care. The physician-to-population ratio is significantly lower in communities with high proportions of racial/ethnic minorities.[30] The absence of nearby primary care facilities may keep those without adequate transportation or family support from seeking care.

Primary health care also may be less affordable for minority youth. Health insurance is central to making health care affordable. Poor adolescents and racial/ethnic minorities are less likely to have insurance.[34,82] A lack of health insurance is associated with fewer doctor visits,[34] and it increases the likelihood of emergency room utilization as a source of nonemergency care.[32] It also acts as a barrier to regular preventive health services such as vaccinations, which are crucial to the prevention of infectious diseases. Other preventive procedures such as mammograms and Pap tests, which aid in the early detection of breast and cervical cancer, are also more accessible to those with health insurance.[2] Furthermore, among insured adolescents, out-of-pocket copayments and the complexity of the health care system may deter socioeconomically disadvantaged families from seeking care.[16]

Confidentiality

Adolescents of all ethnicities need to be able to trust that the information exchanged during a medical visit will remain confidential. Informed consent and payment plans that involve parents are two barriers to confidential care.[3] Many physicians caring for adolescents recognize the need to deliver confidential services. However, physicians may fail to realize that the need for confidentiality may be stronger in some cultures than others. In one study, white adolescents were far more concerned about their parents finding out about their health concerns and behaviors than were adolescents in other racial/ethnic groups.[11] As such, it may be more appropriate, in some instances, for physicians to include parents in the management of their minority adolescent patients' sensitive problems, such as STDs and pregnancy.

Quality of Care

Two perspectives for evaluating quality of care are the patients' and the health care systems'. Patient satisfaction is a measure of the quality of care received. Studies suggest that the manner and style in which care is delivered affects patient satisfaction.[33] Given that there may be cultural and socioeconomic differences between providers and their racial/ethnic minority adolescent patients, potential exists for patient dissatisfaction in the way care is delivered. Patient dissatisfaction may result in the decision not to follow providers' recommendations, which in some instances may compromise the health of the adolescent.

Another measure of the quality of care is whether patients receive necessary and appropriate advice and treatment as determined by the health care system. Although little research pertains specifically to adolescents in this area, several studies have illustrated that cardiovascular procedures are used disproportionately for white adults compared with black adults after controlling for severity of illness.[18,19,35,56,68,80] These studies suggest that there may be a difference in the way doctors make recommendations to their patients based on the patients' race/ethnicity.

Cultural Competency

Culturally determined health-related beliefs and values of patients affect their interpretation and labeling of illness and their decisions about when and where to seek care. In addition, cultural differences between clinicians and their patients may influence the type of information disclosed to the provider, the degree of mutual understanding about a problem, patient acceptance of management plans, and patient satisfaction with the visit. Given that most providers are from cultures different from their racial/ethnic minority patients,[49] physicians must make an effort to deliver primary care that is culturally competent.[69] *Culturally competent primary care* refers to the awareness of the health-related beliefs and values of patients and the integration of these cultural beliefs and values into practice.[13]

The primary health care system currently is not totally culturally competent. There is little diversity among health professionals, and most providers may not provide care in a culturally competent manner.[13,14,69,70] Furthermore, because of the dearth of racial/ethnic minority health care professionals in leadership roles, institutional and professional guidelines and organizational structures may be developed that conflict with the cultures and socioeconomic characteristics of racial/ethnic minority patients.

The low percentage of minority physicians is likely to persist. As recently as 1993, racial/ethnic minorities represented only 10% of all medical students in the United States.[49] One primary factor contributing to the underrepresentation is that minority adolescents are not getting the type of education necessary for entrance to a medical school. In 1992, only 3201 African Americans earned bachelor's degrees in the sciences—the type of degree held by more than two-thirds of medical school enrollees. A secondary problem is that the minorities who do attend medical school report experiencing varying amounts of racial discrimination, both from faculty and fellow students, which may account in part for higher drop-out rates.[8]

Coordination and Comprehensiveness

Minority adolescents may have different and more complex health needs than white adolescents because of factors associated with the neighborhoods in which they live and their lower socioeconomic position. They may demand more comprehensive packages of services, including educational and social services. Given that primary care physicians may be the first to recognize the special needs of these youth, they are often called on to coordinate the services. Insufficient training of physicians in adolescent health care and inadequate funding to reimburse physicians for coordinating these services may limit physicians' abilities to provide coordinated comprehensive primary care.

CONCLUSIONS

Data show that racial/ethnic minority adolescents are less healthy than white, non-Hispanic adolescents. Factors such as low socioeconomic position and neighborhood segregation and factors associated with minority race/ethnicity are associated with worse health status. Combined with the lack of cultural competency among health providers, these factors may contribute to lower quality primary care for minority youth. Efforts to combat the structural inequalities are necessary and should be promoted by health care professionals. In addition, initiatives to increase diversity among physicians and to improve physicians' training in culturally specific health values may increase the quality of care delivered to minority youth. Finally, perhaps most importantly, better data are needed that directly examine the independent role of race/ethnicity, socioeconomic position, environment, and culture on adolescent health to guide efforts to improve the health status of minority adolescents.

References

1. Adler NE, Boyce WT, Chesney MA, et al: Socioeconomic inequalities in health. JAMA 269:3140–3145, 1993.
2. American Cancer Society: Cancer Facts and Figures for Minority Americans. Atlanta, ACS, 1991.

3. American Medical Association, Council on Scientific Affairs: Confidential health services for adolescents. JAMA 269:1420–1424, 1993.
4. Ammerman SD, Nolden M: Neighborhood-based tobacco advertising targeting adolescents. West J Med 162:514–518, 1995.
5. Blackhall LJ, Murphy ST, Frank G, et al: Ethnicity and attitudes toward patient autonomy. JAMA 274:820–825, 1995.
6. Blendon RJ, Aiken LH, Freeman HE, Corey CR: Access to medical care for black and white Americans: A matter of continuing concern. JAMA 261:278–281, 1989.
7. Brandt AM: Racism and research: The case of the Tuskegee syphilis study. In Leavitt JW, Numbers RL (eds): Sickness and Health in America. Madison, University of Wisconsin Press, 1985.
8. Bullock SC, Houston E: Perceptions of racism by black medical students attending white medical schools. J Natl Med Assoc 79:601–608, 1987.
9. Brunswick AF, Boyle JM, Tarica C: Who sees the black doctor? A study of urban black adolescents. Soc Sci Med 13A:45–56, 1979.
10. Centers for Disease Control: Homicide among young black males in the United States, 1978–1987: Leads from the Morbidity and Mortality Weekly Report. JAMA 265:183–184, 1991.
11. Cheng TL, Savageau JA, Sattler AL, DeWitt TG: Confidentiality in health care: A survey of knowledge, perceptions, and attitudes among high school students. JAMA 269:1404–1407, 1993.
12. Congress EP, Lyons BP: Cultural differences in health beliefs: Implications for social work practice in health care settings. Soc Work Health Care 17:81–96, 1992.
13. Davis BJ, Voegtle KH: Culturally Competent Health Care for Adolescents: A Guide for Primary Care Providers. Chicago, American Medical Association, Department of Adolescent Health, 1993.
14. Fernández RL, Kleinman A: Cultural psychiatry: Theoretical, clinical, and research issues. Psychiatr Clin North Am 189:433–448, 1995.
15. Fishman BM, Bobo L, Kosub K, Womeodu RJ: Cultural issues in serving minority populations: Emphasis on Mexican Americans and African Americans. Am J Med Sci 306:160–166, 1993.
16. Friedman E: Money isn't everything: Non-financial barriers to access. JAMA 271:1535–1538, 1994.
17. Gamble VN: A legacy of distrust: African Americans and medical research. Am J Prev Med 9(6 suppl): 35–38, 1993.
18. Gemson DH, Elinson J, Messeri P: Differences in physician prevention practice patterns for white and minority patients. J Commun Health 13:53–64, 1988.
19. Gornick ME, Eggers PW, Reilly TW, et al: Effects of race and income on mortality and use of services among medicare beneficiaries. N Engl J Med 335:791–799, 1996.
20. Lee C: Beyond toxic wastes and race. In Bullard R (ed): Confronting Environmental Racism: Voices from the Grass Roots. Boston, South End Press, 1993, pp 41–52.
21. Krieger N, Wolff MS, Hiatt RA, et al: Breast cancer and serum organochlorines: A prospective study among white, black, and Asian women. J Natl Cancer Inst 86:589–599, 1994.
22. Hackbarth DP, Silvestri B, Cosper W: Tobacco and alcohol billboards in 50 Chicago neighborhoods: Market segmentation to sell dangerous products to the poor. J Public Health Policy 16:213–230, 1995.
23. Hoppe SK, Heller PL: Alienation, familism, and the utilization of health services by Mexican Americans. J Health Soc Behav 16:304–314, 1975.
24. Hummer RA: Black-white differences in health and mortality: A review and conceptual model. Soc Q 37:105–125, 1996.
25. Humphrey DC: Dissection and discrimination: The social origins of cadavers in America, 1760–1915. Bull N Y Acad Med 49:819–827, 1973.
26. Irwin CE Jr, Millstein SG, Ellen JM: Appointment-keeping behavior in adolescents: Factors associated with follow-up appointment-keeping. Pediatrics 92:20–23, 1993.
27. Jones D: African-American clients: Clinical practice issues. Soc Work 24:112–118, 1979.
28. Klein JD, Slap GB, Elster AB, Schonberg SK: Access to health care for adolescents. A position paper of the Society for Adolescent Medicine. J Adolesc Health 13:162–170, 1992.
29. Kleinman A, Eisenberg L, Good B: Culture, illness, and care: Clinical lessons from anthropologic and cross-cultural research. Ann Intern Med 88:251–258, 1978.
30. Komoramy M, Grumbach K, Drak M, et al: The role of Black and Hispanic physicians in providing health care for underserved populations. N Engl J Med 334:1305–1310, 1996.
31. Krieger N, Rowley DL, Herman AA, et al: Racism, sexism, and social class: Implications for studies of health, disease, and well-being. Am J Prev Med 9(6 suppl):82–122, 1993.
32. Lehmann CU, Barr J, Kelly PJ: Emergency department utilization by adolescents. J Adolesc Health 15:485–490, 1994.
33. Levy DR: White doctors and black patients: Influence of race on the doctor-patient relationship. Pediatrics 75:639–643, 1985.

34. Lieu TA, Newachek PW, McManus MA: Race, ethnicity, and access to ambulatory care among US adolescents. Am J Public Health 83:960–965, 1993.
35. Lowe ML, Kerridge IH, Mitchell KR: "These sorts of people don't do very well": Race and allocation of health care resources. J Med Ethics 21:356–360, 1995.
36. Magaña A, Clark NM: Examining a paradox: Does religiosity contribute to positive birth outcomes in Mexican American populations? Health Educ Q 22:96–109, 1995.
37. Markides KS, Coreil J: The health of Hispanics in the Southwestern United States: An epidemiologic paradox. Public Health Rep 101:253–265, 1986.
38. Marmot MG, Smith GD, Stanesfeld S, et al: Health inequalities among British civil servants: The Whitehall II study. Lancet 337:1387–1393, 1987.
39. Massey DS, Eggers ML: The ecology of inequality: Minorities and the concentration of poverty, 1970–1980. Am J Sociol 95:1153–1188, 1990.
40. McKenzie JL, Chrisman NJ: Healing herbs, gods, and magic: Folk health beliefs among Filipino-Americans. Nurs Outlook 25:326–329, 1977.
41. Montgomery LE, Kiely JL, Pappas GP: The effects of poverty, race, and family structure on US children's health: Data from the NHIS, 1978–1980 and 1989–1991. Am J Public Health 86:1401–1405, 1996.
42. Moore DJ, Williams JD, Qualls WJ: Target marketing of tobacco and alcohol-related products to ethnic minority groups in the United States. Ethn Dis 6:83–98, 1996.
43. Moy E, Bartman BA: Physician race and care of minority and medically indigent patients. JAMA 273:1515–1520, 1995.
44. National Center for Health Statistics: Advance report of final mortality statistics, 1994. Monthly vital statistics report; 45(3), suppl. Hyattsville, MD, NCHS, 1996.
45. National Center for Health Statistics: Current estimates from the National Health Interview Survey. Hyattsville, MD, 1991, NCHS Series 10, No. 184.
46. Needleman HL, Schell A, Bellinger D, et al: The long-term effects of exposure to low doses of lead in childhood: An 11-year follow-up report. N Engl J Med 322:83–88, 1990.
47. Newacheck PW, McManus MA: Health insurance status of adolescents in the United States. Pediatrics 84:699–708, 1989.
48. Nickens HW: The health status of minority populations in the United States. West J Med 155:27–32, 1991.
49. Nickens HW, Ready TP, Petersdorf RG: Project 3000 by 2000: Racial and ethnic diversity in US medical schools. N Engl J Med 331:472–476, 1994.
50. Nilchaikovit T, Hill JM, Holland JC: The effects of culture on illness behavior and medical care: Asian and American differences. Gen Hosp Psychiatry 15:41–50, 1993.
51. Oliver ML, Shapiro TS: Black wealth/white wealth: A new perspective on racial inequality. New York, Routledge, 1995.
52. Ozer EM, Brindis CD, Millstein SG, et al: America's Adolescents: Are They Healthy? San Francisco, University of California, National Adolescent Health Information Center, 1997.
53. Pappas G, Queen S, Hadden W, Fisher G: The increasing disparity in mortality between socioeconomic groups in the United States, 1960 and 1986. N Engl J Med 329:103–109, 1993.
54. Parken M: Culture and preventive health care. JOGN Nurs 7(6):40–46, 1978.
55. Penn NE, Kar S, Kramer J, et al: Ethnic minorities, health care systems, and behavior. Health Psychol 14:641–646, 1995.
56. Peterson ED, Shaw LK, DeLong ER, et al: Racial variation in the use of coronary-revascularization procedures: Are the differences real? Do they matter? N Engl J Med 336:480–486, 1997.
57. Quesada GM, Heller PL: Sociocultural barriers to medical care among Mexican Americans in Texas. Med Care 15(5):93–101, 1977.
58. Rubel AJ: The epidemiology of a folk illness: *Susto* in Hispanic America. In Martínez RA (ed): Hispanic Culture in Health Care. St. Louis, Mosby, 1978.
59. Ryan AS: Cultural factors in casework with Chinese-Americans. Soc Casework 66:333–340, 1985.
60. Savitt TL: The use of blacks for medical experimentation and demonstration in the old south. J South Hist 48:331–348, 1982.
61. Schubiner H, Scott R, Tzelepis A: Exposure to violence among inner-city youth. J Adolesc Health 14:214–219, 1993.
62. Scott BM, Denniston RW, Magruder KM: Alcohol advertising in the African-American community. J Drug Iss 22:455–469, 1992.
63. Sells CW, Blum RW: Morbidity and mortality among US adolescents: An overview of data and trends. Am J Public Health 86:513–519, 1996.
64. Shea S, Fullilove MT: Entry of black and other minority students into US medical schools. N Engl J Med 313:933–940, 1985.

65. da Silva GC: Awareness of Hispanic cultural issues in the health care setting. Child Health Care 13:4–10, 1984.
66. Snow LF: Traditional health beliefs and practices among lower class black Americans. West J Med 139:820–828, 1983.
67. Sorlie P, Rogot E, Anderson R, et al: Black-white mortality differences by family income. Lancet 340:346–350, 1992.
68. Stein JA, Fox SA, Murata PJ: The influence of ethnicity, socioeconomic status, and psychological barriers on use of mammography. J Health Soc Behav 32:101–113, 1991.
69. Sue DW, Sue D: Counseling the Culturally Different. New York, Wiley & Sons, 1990.
70. Uba L: Cultural barriers to health care for Southeast Asian refugees. Public Health Rep 107:544–548, 1992.
71. United States Bureau of the Census: Current Population Reports. Washington, DC, P60-189, 1996.
72. United States Bureau of the Census: Current Population Reports. Washington, DC, P25-1095, 1996.
73. United States Bureau of the Census: Household wealth and asset ownership: 1988. Washington, DC, US Government Printing Office, 1990.
74. United States Bureau of the Census: US Census of the Population, US Summary, PC80-1-C1, 1996 and Current Population Reports P20-455, P20-459, P20-462, P20-465RV, P20-475. Washington, DC, 1996.
75. United States Bureau of Labor Statistics: Bulletin 2307. Washington, DC, 1996.
76. United States Department of Commerce, Economics and Statistics Administration: Current Population Reports: Population Projections of the United States by Age, Sex, Race and Hispanic Origin: 1995 to 2050. Washington, DC, Bureau of the Census, 1996.
77. United States Department of Health and Human Services: Cigarette advertising—United States, 1988. MMWR 39:261–265, 1990.
78. Weitzman M, Gortmaker S, Sobol A: Racial, social, and environmental risks for childhood asthma. Am J Dis Child 144:1189–1194, 1990.
79. While D, Kelly S, Huang W, Charlton A: Cigarette advertising and onset of smoking in children: Questionnaire survey. BMJ 313:398–399, 1996.
80. Whittle J, Conigliaro J, Good CB, Lofgren RP: Racial differences in the use of invasive cardiovascular procedures in the department of veterans affairs medical system. N Engl J Med 329:621–627, 1993.
81. Williams DR, Collins C: US socioeconomic and racial differences in health: Patterns and explanations. Annu Rev Sociol 21:349–386, 1995.
82. Wood DL, Hayward RA, Corey CR, et al: Access to medical care for children and adolescents in the United States. Pediatrics (86):666–673, 1990.

Acculturation Issues in Adolescent Immigrants: How Are They Related to Health?

KAREN J. BROWNER-ELHANAN, M.D.

Division of Adolescent Medicine
Montefiore Medical Center
Bronx, New York

Reprint requests to:
Karen J. Browner-Elhanan, M.D.
Division of Adolescent Medicine
Montefiore Medical Center
111 E. 210th Street
Bronx, NY 10470

For adolescents, immigration to a new country is characterized by seemingly insurmountable challenges, including the learning of a new language, assimilation into a strange educational system, and the struggle to develop a new circle of friends. At the same time, the adolescent must deal with the normal intergenerational conflicts characteristic of this stage of development. Difficulty accessing educational, preventive, and primary care medical services is a problem immigrant youth may share with their native peers; however, it may be heightened by cultural barriers, unfamiliarity, and a simple lack of understanding of availability of services.

In addition, health care providers and educators working with immigrant youth may be unfamiliar with, or insensitive to, problems the adolescents may have faced prior to their arrival or during their "settling in" period. Because of this lack of expertise, needed services may not be offered even when they are available.

Many immigrant adolescents have been tortured or witnessed the torture of loved ones. Many more have suffered severe deprivation in refugee camps or transiently during their migration to the new land. These difficulties may cause problems of posttraumatic stress disorder, depression, anxiety, or psychosomatic complaints. In addition, typical cross-generational problems between youth and parents may be exacerbated. This chapter reviews health-related issues of immigrant adolescents from the perspective of the family, the adolescents' mental health, and their physical health.

FAMILY ISSUES

The report of the New York Task Force on Immigrant Health states: "Immigrant adolescents may particularly fear parental reactions to their seeking care that may not be congruent with traditional health practices or conflict with cultural attitudes about gender roles and health behaviors."[13] Adolescents and young adults generally assimilate more quickly than their immigrant parents. They usually learn the new language much more rapidly and learn to identify with different cultural symbols more easily as they develop a new peer group at school. However, if the parents are depressed and demoralized due to the stress of migration, it may be more difficult for the adolescent to adjust to a new social circle. The adolescent's adjustment problems, in turn, may cause the parent to become more depressed and demoralized.[16] It is into this cycle that medical and mental health providers often enter, offering options for services to facilitate adaptation and assimilation.

The clinician must recognize that many of the family problems involving immigrant adolescents are related to the parents' low self-esteem and lack of confidence in their parenting skills. Rotenberg and colleagues state: "When children and adolescents sense despair and a lack of confidence in their parents, they feel themselves insufficiently protected and supported. Tension and aggression frequently appear. The anger may seem as if it is directed against the parents; in fact, it is a reaction to parental weakness. It reflects the adolescent's fear of the future and his inability to accept his parent's passivity."[16] However, parents do not usually recognize the true source of such aggressive behavior, and they begin to quarrel with the adolescent. These battles often serve to emphasize to the adolescent the parents' weakened state of competence. Another cycle develops: both sides become increasingly hostile and aggressive, both toward each other and toward others. The relationship between immigrant parents' low self-esteem and inappropriate reactions of their teenage children has been well-described.[15,16]

When children enter adolescence, new demands are placed on immigrant parents. Often these demands require modifications in more traditional parenting approaches that previously had been accepted by the child. Hattar-Pollara and Meleis describe the experience of the changing approach to parenthood of Jordanian immigrant mothers in the western United States.[6] The mothers describe a constant need to try to balance their desire for their teenagers to maintain an "old country" ethnic identity, while appreciating their need and desire to become acculturated in the receiving community. The youngsters' responses to this struggle vary but often may be volatile.

It becomes evident from these studies that assessment and treatment of parents may be as important to the eventual satisfactory acculturation of immigrant adolescents as is individual treatment. This mandate, however, puts large demands on the health care system in the receiving country because of language and cultural barriers.

MENTAL HEALTH ISSUES OF ADOLESCENTS

Psychological problems associated with immigrant youth can be attributed to poverty, immigration stress caused by homesickness or slow language and cultural adaptation, or posttraumatic stress disorder (PTSD).[11] When traumatic events affect individuals within the child's own nuclear family, the more serious disorders such as PTSD may become evident. Social history shows that after the Blitz in London, during times of conflict in Northern Ireland,[10] and during Arab-Israeli conflicts decades ago,[14] as well as during modern repressive regimes, the risk of psychiatric illness in older children and teenagers exposed to traumatic sights such as bombings was much higher in those to whom personal harm was done or whose loved ones were harmed. Risk of psychosomatic illness was also higher in children who were separated from their parents.

In adolescents, behavior may become aggressive. Sleep problems, conduct disorders, and school failures occur frequently. A study conducted in Israel showed that one-third of 25 Israeli youth whose fathers were killed in war had increased aggressiveness and disciplinary problems and more frequent acute medical conditions 2–3 years after their fathers' deaths compared with previously.[3] Chilean youth resettling in Sweden showed frequent symptoms of PTSD. Of those whose parents had been persecuted, 75% complained of severe sleep disturbances and 50% had depression.[8] Immigration and its frequent accompaniments of economic problems, homelessness, and severe family dysfunction compound previous traumatic life events and may exacerbate the adolescents' anxiety and behavioral disturbances.

Recent studies have compared the "symptom profiles" of Latin American and Southeast Asian immigrant youth in North America.[11,12] Both groups represent large parts of the immigrant population in the United States and Canada. In these cultures studied during the early 1990s, if the family was intact and if minimal personal harm was done to the adolescent or his family, fewer psychosocial and medical problems persisted during the resettlement period. Distinct differences were found to exist, however, between the two groups of immigrant youth. While both Latin American and Southeast Asian immigrant youth suffered from a relatively high rate of PTSD, behavioral problems such as aggression, violent behavior, hyperactivity, and school problems were much more frequent in Latin American youth than in Southeast Asian teenagers. The Asian youths were more likely to withdraw socially yet remain motivated in school relative to their Latino peers. These differences, however, may be due to the unique effects of war on youth and may not be directly related to the stress of immigration and acculturation. Violent political upheavals and domestic violence in Central American and Mexican families were found to profoundly influence youth, and were significantly associated with PTSD. In contrast, studies from the late 1980s about the effects of massive trauma on Cambodian children showed a comparatively lower rate of conduct disorders and aggressive behavior.[18] Davanzo interviewed young Cambodian women and described their coping strategies and different manifestations of acculturation, among which somatic symptoms were the most common complaint.[2]

These studies present a clear picture of a group of psychosocial problems that the provider working with adolescents should look for and assess in a new immigrant patient. Symptoms include depression and social withdrawal, depression and school failure, and acting out. An evaluation of risk factors includes assessing whether the family is intact and whether the youth or family have experienced personal trauma. In addition, it is important to assess whether the parents are depressed and lacking self-esteem due to past traumatic experiences or strains of immigration and are thus unable to provide adequate support to their adolescent child.

Other social support systems also should be investigated and evaluated. Studies of adopted children and studies of adaptation of refugees show that cultural adaptation for everyone, especially youth, is smoother and simpler if there is ethnic and cultural similarity within the new environment.[9] The link to the familiar past helps the new immigrant to adapt to his new "global community." Thus, the positive aspects of teen gang associations and gang activity within immigrant communities in North America, particularly in large urban areas, include a strong culturally appropriate support network and rich, health-promoting, socializing opportunities. Although these gangs are often perceived as antisocial and promoting violent conflicts, they may actually, with the support network they provide, ameliorate many adaptation problems that immigrant youth face.

They may serve as an adjunct to the role that schools and medical facilities play in helping youth adapt to their new environment.[13]

PHYSICAL HEALTH ISSUES OF ADOLESCENTS

In addition to mental health problems, health care providers need to be familiar with the physical health needs of young immigrants. Fitzpatrick et al. reported that 52% of a group of new Southeast Asian immigrant teenagers in San Diego had positive PPD skin tests, 39% lacked immunizations, 35% had positive stool specimens for parasites, 14% had positive tests for hepatitis B antigen, 8% were chronic carriers of hepatitis B, 10% were anemic, and 19% had hemoglobinopathies.[4] In addition, 14% were below the fifth percentile for both height and weight, 12% had goiter, 12% had skin disorders, 5% had a hearing loss, and 4% had idiopathic scoliosis as diagnosed on a routine physical examination. Other illnesses that are common among Asian immigrant youth include infectious diseases, primarily parasitic intestinal and skin infections, upper respiratory infections with sore throats, and otitis media.[1] Incomplete immunizations and malnutrition are also common among other ethnic groups of young immigrants. Parasites causing intestinal malabsorption, respiratory tract infections, and chronic otitis media, including otitis media that causes hearing loss, are widespread in immigrant adolescents in cities throughout the world.

Uniken Venema found that a group of 15-year-old Surinamese and Moroccan teenagers living in the Netherlands were significantly less likely to rate their own health as good than Dutch children of the same age, gender, and educational background.[19] The study also found that Turkish and Surinamese youth in the same area reported many more psychosomatic complaints than their Dutch neighbors despite a similar rate of reported chronic physical illnesses among the groups.

An increased risk of testing positive on PPD skin tests was highly associated with being foreign-born among students in schools in a suburb of Toronto.[17] Ten refugee children from Somalia were diagnosed with active tuberculosis, which prompted Canadian health officers to recommend that foreign-born students be screened for tuberculosis upon school registration. Such school-related screening is also recommended in many states in the United States where the immigrant population is rapidly growing.

Screening of young immigrants for human immunodeficiency virus (HIV) infection is a more difficult issue, and the benefits are less clear than for tuberculosis. The absolute number of HIV-infected immigrant youth is increasing. Screening would identify infected youth and provide insight into their acculturation process as well as facilitate their referral to specialized medical and social services.[5] Hingson and coworkers anonymously surveyed 3049 middle and high school students in Boston about their knowledge of HIV and methods of prevention.[7] Fewer than 40% of sexually active foreign-born high school students reported using condoms, and 4% reported having intercourse with users of intravenous drugs, compared with greater than 60% and 1%, respectively, of their nonimmigrant peers. The researchers concluded that AIDS education must be taught to immigrant students in their native language.[9]

Associations between immigrant status and risk behavior patterns and how these patterns influence health practices and health status in adolescents are important issues for health providers. Velez and Ungemack studied the role of psychological variables that might explain the processes by which Puerto Rican youth become more vulnerable to drug use and addiction after emigration to New York City.[20] Puerto Rican youngsters who had been in New York City longer were more likely to report few parental controls and to have friends who used illicit drugs as additional risk factors to their own drug use. The Puerto Rican adolescent's generational status was clearly associated with different patterns of psychosocial risk factors for illicit drug use. Illicit drug use was far more prevalent among the immigrant youth in New York than among their peers in Puerto Rico.

SUMMARY

Surveying and assessing mental and physical health data among different groups of immigrant adolescents elucidates specific behavioral and physical sequelae. The spectrum of infectious and chronic diseases, as well as critical mental health issues such as PTSD, intergenerational conflict, and risk behaviors have been described. Service providers, health policy makers, and planners need to continue the effort to better understand the characteristics of each adolescent immigrant population to be able to responsibly address the medical and psychosocial needs of these youth and their families.

References

1. Dashefsky B, Teele D: Infectious disease problems in Indochinese refugees. Pediatr Ann 12:232–244, 1983.
2. D'Avanzo CE, Frye B, Froman R: Stress in Cambodian refugee families. Image 26:101–105, 1994.
3. Elizur E, Kaffman M: Children's bereavement reactions following death of the father. J Am Acad Child Psychiatry 21:474–480, 1982.
4. Fitzpatrick S, Johnson J, Shragg P, Felice M: Health care needs of Indochinese refugees. Pediatrics 79:118–124, 1987.
5. Gallagher MA: Human immunodeficiency virus and immigration status in the United States. J Assoc Nurses AIDS Care 3(2):32–35, 1992.
6. Hattar-Pollara M, Meleis AI: Parenting their adolescents: The experiences of Jordanian immigrant women in California. Health Care Women Int 16(3):195–211, 1995.
7. Hingson RW, Strunin L, Grady M, et al: Knowledge about HIV and behavioral risks of foreign-born Boston public school students. Am J Public Health 81:1638–1641, 1991.
8. Hjern A, Angel B, Hofer B: Persecution and Behavior: A report on refugee children from Chile. Child Abuse Negl 15:239–248, 1991.
9. Lin-Fu JS: Population characteristics and health care needs of Asian Pacific Americans. Public Health Rep 103:18–27, 1988.
10. Lyons HA: Psychiatric sequelae of the Belfast riots. Br J Psychiatry 118:265–273, 1971.
11. McCloskey LA, Southwick K: Psychosocial problems in refugee children exposed to war. Pediatrics 97:394–397, 1996.
12. McCloskey LA, Southwick K, Fernandez-Esquer ME, Locke C: A comparative study of the psychological effects of political and domestic violence on Central American and Mexican immigrant mothers and children. J Commun Psychol 16:101–123, 1982.
13. New York Task Force on Immigrant Health, New York University School of Medicine: Roundtable Discussion Notes: Health and adolescent immigrants in New York. New York, NYU School of Medicine, October and December 1991.
14. Punamaki RL, Suleiman R: Predictors and effectiveness of coping with political violence among Palestinian children. Br J Soc Psychol 118:265–273, 1971.
15. Ritsner M, Ponizofsky A, Ginath Y: Demoralization among Russian immigrants: Three years following immigration. Research Report Talpieth Mental Health, 1993.
16. Rotenberg V, Tobin M, Krause D, Lubovkov I: Psychosocial problems faced during absorption of Russian-speaking new immigrants into Israel: A systematic approach. Isr J Psychiatry Relat Sci 3:40–49, 1996.
17. Rothman LM, Dubeski G: School contact tracing following a cluster of tuberculosis cases in two Scarborough schools. Can J Public Health 84:297–302, 1993.
18. Sack WH, Angell RH, Kinzie JD, Rath B: The psychiatric effects of massive trauma on Cambodian children: II. J Am Acad Child Psychiatry 25:3777–3783, 1986.
19. Uniken Venema HP, Garretsen HFL, Van der Maas PJ: Health of migrants and migrant health policy: the Netherlands as an example. Soc Sci Med 41:809–818, 1995.
20. Velez CN, Ungemack JA: Psychosocial correlates of drug use among Puerto Rican youth: Generational status differences. Soc Sci Med 40:91–103, 1995.

"Sex, Drugs, Rock 'n' Roll," and the Media—Are the Media Responsible for Adolescent Behavior?

VICTOR C. STRASBURGER, M.D.

Professor of Pediatrics
Chief, Division of Adolescent Medicine
University of New Mexico School of Medicine
Albuquerque, New Mexico

Reprint requests to:
Victor C. Strasburger, M.D.
Professor of Pediatrics
Chief, Division of Adolescent Medicine
University of New Mexico School of Medicine
Albuquerque, NM 87131

> If parents could package psychological influences to administer in regular doses to their children, I doubt that many would deliberately select Western gunslingers, hopped-up psychopaths, deranged sadists, slap-stick buffoons and the like, unless they entertained rather peculiar ambitions for their growing offspring. Yet such examples of behavior are delivered in quantity, with no direct charge, to millions of households daily. Harried parents can easily turn off demanding children by turning on a television set; as a result, today's youth is being raised on a heavy dosage of televised aggression and violence.
>
> —TV researcher Albert Bandura[5]

One of the most interesting and crucial questions of the 1990s is: What role do the media play in the major adolescent morbidities of sex (teenage pregnancy, sexually transmitted diseases), drugs, and violence (homicide, suicide, interpersonal aggression)? Do television and movies merely reflect a society which is increasingly violent, drug-oriented, and sexualized—as the entertainment industry maintains—or do the media actually *cause* some of the behaviors they depict?

EXPOSURE

Teenagers are inundated with media of all sorts, from television and movies to video games and the Internet. Nielsen data (Table 1) show that American teenagers view about 3 hours of television per day,[1] making it the preeminent medium and exposing the average teenager annually to:

TABLE 1. Time Spent Watching Television in the United States

Age Group	Time Spent Watching Television (hours:minutes/week)
2- to 11-year-olds	23:01
12- to 17-year olds	21:50
18+ year-old men	30:41
18+ year-old women	34:57
55+ year-old men	38:47
55+ year-old women	44:11

From AC Nielsen Company: Nielsen Report on Television 1992–1993. New York, Nielsen Media Research, 1993.

- 10,000 acts of violence,[47]
- 15,000 sexual innuendoes, jokes, and behaviors,[41] and
- 20,000 commercials, including 1,000–2,000 beer and wine advertisements.[70]

Although children and teenagers do not watch as much TV as adults, they are uniquely vulnerable to its effects. Movies tend to be more violent, sexually explicit, and graphic in terms of drug use, but teenagers do not spend an average of 22 hours per week going to the local cinema.

Violence

In the past 2 years, new content analyses of television have caused increased concern among parents and health professionals. In 1996, Mediascope completed its first year of the most comprehensive examination of American television ever undertaken, the National Television Violence Study, which documented that primetime television is not only violent but contains unhealthy messages about violence and conflict resolution (Table 2).[56] A second 1996 study found small decreases in network programming violence from 1994, but the study has many methodologic flaws and was funded by the networks themselves.[16] Finally, a recent comprehensive analysis of rock music videos of all genres demonstrated that 22.4% of all Music Television (MTV) videos portrayed overt violence, 20% of all rap videos contained violence, and 25% of all MTV videos depicted weapon carrying.[30]

Sex

Four recent Kaiser Foundation studies have examined sexual content in current television programming, with the following conclusions: (1) sexual activity is one of the leading topics of discussion on TV talk shows;[39] (2) soap operas contain an average of 6.1 sexual behaviors per hour (unchanged from 1994) but only 10% of them involve discussions of birth control or consequences of sexual activity (Table 3);[43] (3) one-third

TABLE 2. Findings of the National Television Violence Study*

- Overall, 57% of television programming contains violent content.
- The impact of violence is rarely shown, and perpetrators go unpunished in 73% of all violent scenes. Only 4% of violent programs contain antiviolence messages.
- One-fourth of the violent scenes on television involve the use of a handgun.
- For boys ages 10–14, "parental discretion" advisories and PG-13 and R ratings seem to make programs and movies more attractive.

* 2500 hours of programming examined.
Adapted from Mediascope, Inc.: National Television Violence Study. Studio City, CA, Mediascope, 1996.

TABLE 3. Sexual Content of Soap Operas

Behaviors	Number of Behaviors*	Average/Hour
Passionate kissing	165	1.66
Verbal discussions about intercourse	66	0.68
Petting/Caressing	30	0.31
Prostitution	27	0.28
Visual depictions of intercourse	17	0.19
Rape	13	0.14
Discussions of "safe sex," contraception, or AIDS	9	0.09

Adapted from Heintz-Knowles KE: Sexual Activity on Daytime Soap Operas: A Content Analysis of Five Weeks of Television Programming. Menlo Park, CA, Kaiser Family Foundation, 1996.
* 97 hours of programming reviewed.

of teenagers believe that movies and television portray teens having sexual intercourse as normal; teenagers also state that the media are one of the leading sources of sex information for them (Table 4);[64] and (4) the so-called "family hour" of primetime television (8–9 p.m.) contains more than eight sexual incidents per hour, more than four times as much as in 1976.[51]

Drugs

A 1994 study of the 62 top-grossing films from 1960–1990 found that levels of smoking remained constant despite decreases in real life and that lead characters were far more likely to smoke on screen (65%) than their real-life counterparts with similar demographic characteristics.[42,50] Similarly, an American Lung Association study of 133 movies released in 1994–95 found that 77% depicted tobacco use.[78] Cigars also seem to be making a major comeback; more than half of American films now feature them.[78] In other words, Hollywood sometimes does a poor job of "mirroring" society (Table 5).

Advertising of cigarettes and alcohol products remains problematic as well. Tobacco manufacturers spend an estimated $6 billion a year on advertising, and the alcohol industry spends $2 billion a year.[73] Although both industries dispute the notion that they are pitching their wares to teenagers, their choice of advertising stars (e.g., frogs and party dogs) and several studies draw opposite conclusions (Tables 6 and 7).

While smoking and drinking are commonplace in movies, they remain relatively less common on network TV, especially smoking. Only 2% of series stars smoke on TV.[70] However, TV characters rarely refuse to smoke or express antismoking sentiments—probably so as not to offend the corporate advertisers whose parent companies also own tobacco subsidiaries.[67]

TABLE 4. Sources of Sexual Information for Teenagers

Source	%
Teachers, school nurses, or classes at school	40%
Media: TV, movies, or magazines	39%
Parents	36%
Peers	27%
Brothers, sisters, or cousins	12%
Physician or nurse	9%

Adapted from Princeton Survey Research Associates: The 1996 Kaiser Family Foundation Survey on Teens and Sex: What They Say Teens Today Need to Know, and Who They Listen to. Menlo Park, CA, Kaiser Family Foundation, 1996.

TABLE 5. Cigarette Smoking in 1996 Feature Movies

Movie	Number of Smoking Incidents
Trees Lounge (R)	43
The Associate (PG-13)	30
High School High (PG-13)	26
Michael Collins (R)	25
The Big Night (R)	25
Dear God (PG)	25
Sleepers (R)	24
Swingers (R)	22
William Shakespeare's Romeo & Juliet (PG-13)	16
That Thing You Do! (PG)	16
The Chamber (R)	16
The First Wives Club (PG)	10

Adapted from Thomas K: Lighting up: Tobacco has a role in most movies. USA Today, November 7, 1996, p 6D.

Certainly, the potential *fuel* is present, but the fact that American media contain a lot of violence, inappropriate sexual behavior, and drug use does not constitute a specific, scientific, cause-and-effect finding. Content analyses are not equipped to handle such questions.[71] Mere exposure may be concerning, but it is not tantamount to greater harm unless there is a direct relationship between viewing and behavior. What evidence is there?

TABLE 6. Is Cigarette Advertising Effective?

Advertising in Millions of Dollars	Adolescent Brand Preference	Adult Brand Preference
1. Marlboro ($75)	1. Marlboro (60.0%)	1. Marlboro (23.5%)
2. Camel ($43)	2. Camel (13.3%)	2. Winston (6.7%)
3. Newport ($35)	3. Newport (12.7%)	3. Newport (4.8%)

From Centers for Disease Control: Changes in the cigarette brand preferences of adolescent smokers—United States, 1989–1993. MMWR 43:577, 1994; and Pollay RW, Siddarth S, Siegel M, et al: The last straw? Cigarette advertising and realized market shares among youth and adults, 1979–1993. J Marketing 50:1, 1996.

TABLE 7. Are the Budweiser Frogs Effective Advertising? Commercial and Character Recall by Children 9–11 Years Old

Character	Slogan or Motto	% Recall (n = 221)
Bugs Bunny	Eh, what's up Doc?	80
Budweiser Frogs	Bud-weis-er	73
Tony the Tiger	They're grrreat!	57
Smokey Bear	Only you can prevent forest fires	43
Mighty Morphin' Power Rangers	It's morphin' time! or Power up!	39

Adapted from Leiber L: Commercial and character slogan recall by children aged 9 to 11 years: Budweiser frogs versus Bugs Bunny. Berkeley, CA, Center on Alcohol Advertising, 1996.

WHAT THE RESEARCH SAYS

Violence

The research is voluminous and very clear on the relationship between media violence and real-life aggression: a cause-and-effect relationship exists.[20,23,27,29,47] Two government reports, the 1972 Surgeon General's Report,[77] and the 1982 National Institute of Mental Health (NIMH)[58] report reached identical conclusions.

As long ago as the 1960s, laboratory experiments by Bandura (whose quote begins this article) established that young children are likely to imitate what they see on the TV screen, particularly if the behavior is performed by an attractive role model and is rewarded or goes unpunished.[7] Several longitudinal correlational studies have tracked children or adults over a period of up to 30 years and found that viewing violence in the media at age 8 years and younger is a significant risk factor for adolescent or adult aggressive behavior or even criminal violence.[8,15,44,46,68,80] Researchers have concluded that children learn their attitudes about violence at a very young age and, once learned, the attitudes tend to be life-long.[32]

American media are also rife with portrayals of *justified violence* (e.g., the "good guy" beating up the "bad guy"), which is the single strongest positive reinforcer for young people.[6,72] As one leading researcher recently noted, "The scientific debate is over."[31] Not only can media violence promote aggressive or antisocial behavior, it may also desensitize viewers to future violence and can increase viewers' perception that they are living in a mean and dangerous world.[20] The problem is that the entertainment industry does not want to admit the connection any more than the tobacco industry will acknowledge a cause-and-effect relationship between cigarette smoking and lung cancer.[15]

Media violence is not the sole cause of violence in society: poverty, racism, inadequate parenting, the dissolution of the American family, and individual psychological differences all may have far more impact. However, media violence is the one factor that could be changed virtually overnight. How much does media violence contribute to real-life violence? When 22 separate estimates of effect size were collated from various surveys, the size of the effect was 5–15%,[22] but this could represent a sizeable underestimate since social science research has great difficulty approximating real life.[72] Interestingly, the entertainment industry is quick to take credit for the ennobling and positive programming it creates (e.g., the movie Schindler's List) but refuses to take responsibility for any negative repercussions of its meaner efforts.

During the past three decades, the suicide rate among adolescents has quadrupled (coinciding with the "golden age" of TV violence).[74] Several studies in the United States and Europe have demonstrated a link between televised portrayals or news reports about suicide and an increase in teenage suicide.[36–38,62,63,65] The mechanism involved may be that a vulnerable teenager identifies with the suicide victim, and the news or portrayal serves as a catalyst for an attempt.[25]

What links adolescent homicides and suicides to American media is the glamorization of guns (Table 8).[20] Homicide and suicide are the second and third leading causes of death among adolescents, and guns contribute significantly to both.[14] Although there are no specific data linking viewing gunplay in the media with actual gun-related offenses, the connection seems logical, at least to one TV critic:[4]

> On average, a violent crime is committed [in the United States] every 17 seconds. The entertainment industry alone cannot be blamed for this, any more than guns alone, and not the people who pull their triggers, can be blamed for gun-related deaths. But the connections are inescapable. If there were fewer guns, fewer people would be shot to death; if there were fewer violent images, fewer people might be moved to seek violent solutions.

TABLE 8. Handguns and American Youth

- The United States leads all industrialized nations in homicides, with four times the next highest rate (9.8 per 100,000).[a,b]
- Firearms are involved in 68–75% of all homicides, mostly handguns.[c] In California, among 15- to 19-year-olds guns account for 90% of all homicides.[d]
- Although Americans say that they are purchasing handguns for protection, guns in the home are 43 times more likely to kill a family member than an intruder.[e]
- Firearm injuries are the third or fourth leading cause of accidental death among children (depending on age and region).[f]
- The United States is the most heavily armed nation, with as many guns as households (200 million).[g]
- Half of adolescent males and nearly one-fourth of adolescent females report that they could easily obtain a handgun if they desired.[h]
- Nearly 8% of students had carried a gun to school during the 30 days prior to the 1995 Youth Risk Behavior Survey.[i]
- The sale of toy guns represents a nearly $100 million industry.[j]
- One-fourth of the violent scenes on television involve use of a handgun.[k]

[a] Fingerhut LA, Kleinman JC: International and interstate comparisons of homicide among young males. JAMA 263:3292–3295, 1990.
[b] 1993 Demographic Yearbook. New York, United Nations, 1995.
[c] Cohall AT, Cohall RM: "Number one with a bullet": Epidemiology and prevention of homicide among adolescents and young adults. Adolesc Med State Art Rev 6:183–197, 1995.
[d] Chu LD, Sorenson SB: Trends in California homicide, 1970 to 1993. West J Med 165:119–125, 1996.
[e] Kellerman AL, Reay DT: Protection or peril? An analysis of firearm-related deaths in the home. N Engl J Med 314:1557–1560, 1986.
[f] Senturia YD, Cristoffel KK, Donovan M: Children's household exposure to guns: A pediatric practice-based survey. Pediatrics 93:469–475, 1994.
[g] Davidson OG: Under Fire: The NRA and the Battle for Gun Control. New York, Holt, 1993.
[h] Callahan CM, Rivara FP: Urban high school youth and handguns: A school-based survey. JAMA 267:3038–3041, 1992.
[i] Centers for Disease Control: Youth Risk Behavior Surveillance—United States, 1995. MMWR 44(SS-4): 1–84, 1996.
[j] Strasburger VC: Television and adolescents: Sex, drugs, rock 'n' roll. Adolesc Med State Art Rev 1: 161–194, 1990.
[k] Mediascope, Inc.: National Television Violence Study. Studio City, CA, Mediascope, 1996.

Sex

Unfortunately, the data are not nearly as clear for the relationship between early sexual activity and a heavy diet of sexualized content in the media. While there are more than 1,000 studies linking media violence to real-life violence, there are only five studies demonstrating any connection between sexy media and changes in teenagers' sexual behavior or attitudes:

- In a study of 75 adolescent girls, half of whom were pregnant, the pregnant girls watched more soap operas before becoming pregnant and were less likely to think that their favorite soap characters would use birth control.[24]
- A study of 391 junior high school students in North Carolina found that those who selectively viewed more sexy TV were more likely to have begun having sexual intercourse in the preceding year.[10]
- A study of 326 Cleveland teenagers showed that those with a preference for MTV had increased amounts of sexual experience in their midteen years.[60]
- Data from the National Surveys of Children revealed that males who watch more TV had the highest prevalence of sexual intercourse and that teens who watched TV apart from their family had a rate of intercourse 3–6 times higher than those who viewed with their family.[61]

• A 1997 study found that young teenagers exposed to more soap operas and talk shows tended to have beliefs consistent with what they were viewing (e.g., "married people often cheat on their husband or wife," "most of my friends have had sex with someone").[75]

Thus, for sexual activity, inferences must be drawn from the violence literature (i.e., if children and teenagers can learn aggressive behavior, why shouldn't they be able to learn sexual behavior?)[12] In addition, the 1985 Guttmacher Report found that the United States has the highest teenage pregnancy rate in the Western world, and the authors speculated this was because American society:[49] (1) refuses to allow easy access to birth control, (2) refuses to allow high quality, comprehensive sex education in schools, and (3) allows inappropriate sexual messages and behaviors to be shown in the media.

Sexual Violence

Considerable research on sexual violence delineates a major impact of explicit depictions of sexual violence on attitudes and beliefs, especially of males.[28,29] Although *any* depiction of violence can result in increased aggression or decreased sensitivity toward women, sexualized violence is particularly suspect.[28,55,57] Only in the United States is eroticism in the media considered more harmful than violence; for the rest of the Western world, the opposite is true.[34] Given the findings in the scientific literature, the rest of the Western world is correct.

Drugs

Studies indicate that $8 billion of advertising that tobacco and alcohol manufacturers pitch every year to the American public have an impact on adolescents' beliefs and attitudes about smoking and drinking. As long as 20 years ago, the National Science Foundation commissioned a report on the effects of advertising on children, which concluded:[59]

> It is clear from the available evidence that television *does* influence children. Research has demonstrated that children attend to and learn from commercials, and that advertising is at least moderately successful in creating positive attitudes toward and the desire for products advertised. . . . Younger viewers . . . appear to be the most vulnerable.

Numerous recent studies document that children and adolescents who are exposed to greater amounts of tobacco or alcohol advertising are more likely to use or intend to use such products.[2,13,33,40,54,70] This makes intuitive sense as well: $8 billion a year is a lot of money to commit to advertising if it does not influence people to consume your product.

WHAT THE RESEARCH DOESN'T SAY

Although the literature on media violence is substantial and so convincing that researchers have stopped doing basic studies, it does not yet yield many solutions. A few studies have examined whether children can be "counter-programmed" to resist media violence. In 1983 researchers developed a curriculum for first- and third-graders that resulted in changing students' attitudes about televised violence and their own level of aggressive behavior as rated by their peers.[45] At Yale, Singer et al. developed a critical viewing curriculum for third- through fifth-graders.[69] Media literacy and critical viewing skills are now viewed as being solutions to the problem, but few curricula have undergone careful scientific scrutiny.

What is also completely unknown is which children or adolescents are most vulnerable to media myths and stereotypes. Research indicates that there is considerable variability in how teenagers view the same program, depending on their ethnicity, family background, and other characteristics.[11]

By contrast, there is a desperate need for more research into the connection between sexual content on television, in the movies, and in rock music and music videos and changes in adolescents' sexual beliefs, attitudes or behavior.[18,21] Is the same causal connection in effect? What factors mitigate against a deleterious effect? Are all children and adolescents equally vulnerable, and is there a "window of vulnerability"? Such research is difficult to do given the intrinsic conservatism of American society, but it is absolutely necessary. In particular, there has never been a large-scale, longitudinal correlational study of heavy media consumption and adolescents' sexual attitudes or behavior.

The advertising-consumption research is convincing regarding children and adolescents, but what is unknown, again, is how to counteract the unhealthy aspects of advertising. In addition, teenagers might be susceptible to antidrug messages embedded creatively in mainstream programming.[9] At present, counteradvertising does not seem able to reach the density that mainstream advertising has, thus making it less useful as a solution.[72]

Finally, far more research is needed regarding adolescent suicide and media portrayals, the influence of rock music and music videos on adolescents,[76] the effects of video games,[35] and the potential connection between eating disorders and the media.[26,52,53]

SOLUTIONS

Although a complete discussion of solutions is beyond the scope of this chapter, a few suggestions might be useful:

• **More research.** Media research is difficult, sometimes tedious, and often expensive. However, considering the significant impact that the media have on young people, more media research is desperately needed, including adequate funding for such efforts. A new NIMH report on television by the year 2000 would also be extremely useful to researchers, health professionals, parents, and policymakers.

• **Less media violence.** Numerous studies show that the American public is appalled at the current levels of violence on television and in movies, but the entertainment industry continues to go about business as usual.[3] The industry continues to minimize its public responsibility and the impact of television and movies on young people.

• **Media literacy programs.** Although improving the quality of programming is a must, children and teenagers must still learn how to decode the subtle and not-so-subtle messages contained in television programming, advertising, movies, and music videos. Parents need to begin this process when their children are 2–3 years old (Table 9), but school programs may be extremely useful as well. The American Academy of Pediatrics is planning to embark on a major campaign to emphasize the need for media literacy.

TABLE 9. Five Important Ideas to Teach Children and Adolescents about Television

1. You are smarter than what you see on TV.
2. TV's world is not real.
3. TV teaches that some people are more important than others.
4. TV keeps doing the same things over and over again.
5. Somebody is always trying to make money with TV.

Adapted from Davis J: Five important ideas to teach your children about TV. Media & Values 59/60:10–14, 1992.

TABLE 10. Questions to Ask When Taking a Media History

- How many hours a day do you watch television?
- How do you decide what shows to watch? Movies?
- Where is (are) the television(s) in your home?
- Are there any "house rules" regarding viewing (e.g., no viewing until all homework is completed)?
- What are your favorite television programs? Movies?
- Are there rules regarding music videos? Video games?
- Who watches television with you?
- Do you "surf" the Internet?

Adapted from American Medical Association: Physician Guide to Media Violence. Chicago, AMA, 1996.

• **A ban on cigarette advertising in all media and a ban on promotional activities aimed at young people (e.g., merchandising, rock concerts), and the restriction of alcohol advertising to "tombstone ads."** American society pays a high price for allowing tobacco manufacturers unlimited access to children and adolescents, and the connection between advertising and consumption is now clearly established. Any product as harmful as tobacco should have severe restrictions placed upon it, including a ban on all advertising. Tombstone ads involve showing the "purity" of the product only, not all of the qualities that the purchaser will supposedly gain by consuming it. Such restrictions have already been endorsed by the Federal Drug Administration, the Surgeon General, the American Academy of Pediatrics, and the American Medical Association.[13,17,79] Because advertising these products represents "commercial speech" and not "free speech," they are not automatically protected under the First Amendment.[48,66]

• **Greater sensitivity on the part of primary care physicians, especially pediatricians and adolescent medicine specialists, to the influence of the media on young people.** Most physicians with adolescent patients are well aware of the influence that peers can have, but they may be completely unaware that television and other media function as a sort of "super-peer." The influence of media needs to be controlled from the outset, since what is learned between ages 2 and 10 may be played out during adolescence with harmful or unhealthy consequences. Therefore, parents of young children need to be counseled to limit their young children's viewing to no more than 1–2 hours per day, to guide their choice of programs, and to view with them.[19] Parents of teenagers need to be familiar with what media choices their teens are making and discuss them frequently and rigorously. Finally, physicians need to learn to take media histories from their patients (Table 10).[3]

References

1. AC Nielsen Company: Nielsen Report on Television 1992–1993. New York, Nielsen Media Research, 1993.
2. Altman DG, Levine DW, Coeytaux R, et al: Tobacco promotion and susceptibility to tobacco use among adolescents aged 12 through 17 years in a nationally representative sample. Am J Public Health 86:1590–1593, 1996.
3. American Medical Association: Physician Guide to Media Violence. Chicago, AMA, 1996.
4. Auletta K: What won't they do? The New Yorker 69:45–73, 1993.
5. Bandura A: What TV violence can do to your child. Look, October 22, 1963, pp 46–52.
6. Bandura A: Influence of models' reinforcement contingencies on the acquisition of imitative responses. J Pers Social Psychol 1:589–595, 1965.
7. Bandura A, Ross D, Ross SA: Imitation of film-mediated aggressive models. J Abnorm Soc Psychol 66:3–11, 1963.

8. Belson WA: Television Violence and the Adolescent Boy. Westmead, UK, Saxon House, Teakfield Ltd., 1978.
9. Borzekowski DLG: Embedded anti-alcohol messages on commercial television: What teenagers perceive. J Adolesc Health 19:345–352, 1996.
10. Brown JD, Newcomer SF: Television viewing and adolescents' sexual behavior. J Homosex 21:77–91, 1991.
11. Brown JD, Schulze L: The effects of race, gender, and fandom on audience interpretations of Madonna's music videos. J Commun 40:88–102, 1990.
12. Brown JD, Steele JR: Sex and the Mass Media. Menlo Park, CA, Kaiser Family Foundation, 1995.
13. Centers for Disease Control: Preventing tobacco use among young people: A report of the Surgeon General. Atlanta, U.S. Department of Health and Human Services, 1994.
14. Centers for Disease Control: Deaths resulting from firearm- and motor-vehicle-related injuries—United States, 1968–1991. MMWR 43:37–42, 1994.
15. Centerwall BS: Television and violence: The scale of the problem and where to go from here. JAMA 267:3059–3063, 1992.
16. Cole J: The UCLA Television Violence Report 1996. Los Angeles: UCLA Center for Communication Policy, 1996.
17. Committee on Communications, American Academy of Pediatrics: Children, adolescents and advertising [policy statement]. Pediatrics 95:295–297, 1995.
18. Committee on Communications, American Academy of Pediatrics: Adolescent sexuality and the media [policy statement]. Pediatrics 95:298–300, 1995.
19. Committee on Communications, American Academy of Pediatrics: Children, adolescents, and television [policy statement]. Pediatrics 96:786–787, 1995.
20. Committee on Communications, American Academy of Pediatrics: Media violence [policy statement]. Pediatrics 95:949–951, 1995.
21. Committee on Communications, American Academy of Pediatrics: Impact of music lyrics and music videos on children and youth [policy statement]. Pediatrics 98:1219–1221, 1996.
22. Comstock G, Strasburger VC: Deceptive appearances: Television violence and aggressive behavior—An introduction. J Adolesc Health Care 11:31–44, 1990.
23. Comstock G, Strasburger VC: Media violence: Q & A. Adolesc Med State Art Rev 4:495–509, 1993.
24. Corder-Bolz C: Television and adolescents' sexual behavior. Sex Education Coalition News 3:40, 1981.
25. Davidson LE, Rosenberg ML, Mercy JA, et al: An epidemiologic study of risk factors in two teenage suicide clusters. JAMA 262:2687–2692, 1989.
26. Dietz WH: Television, obesity, and eating disorders. Adolesc Med State Art Rev 4:543–549, 1993.
27. Dietz WH, Strasburger VC: Children, adolescents, and television. Curr Probl Pediatr 21:8–31, 1991.
28. Donnerstein E, Linz D: Sexual violence in the mass media. In Costanzo M, Oskamp S (eds): Violence and the Law. Newbury Park, CA, Sage, 1994, pp 9–36.
29. Donnerstein E, Linz D: The mass media: A role in injury causation and prevention. Adolesc Med State Art Rev 6:271–284, 1995.
30. DuRant RH, Rich M, Emans SJ, et al: Violence and weapon carrying in music videos: A content analysis. Arch Pediatr Adolesc Med 151:443–448, 1997.
31. Eron LR: The Problem of Media Violence and Children's Behavior. New York, Guggenheim Foundation, 1993.
32. Eron LR: Media violence. Pediatr Ann 24:84–87, 1995.
33. Evans N, Farkas A, Gilpin E, et al: Influence of tobacco marketing and exposure to smokers on adolescent susceptibility to smoking. J Natl Cancer Inst 87:1538–1545, 1995.
34. Federman J: Media Ratings: Design, Use and Consequences. Studio City, CA, Mediascope, 1996.
35. Funk J, Buchman DD: Video game controversies. Pediatr Ann 24:91–94, 1995.
36. Gould MS, Davidson L: Suicide contagion among adolescents. Adv Adolesc Ment Health 3:29–59, 1988.
37. Gould MS, Shaffer D: The impact of suicide in television movies. N Engl J Med 315:690–694, 1986.
38. Gould MS, Shaffer D, Kleinman M: The impact of suicide in television movies: Replication and commentary. Suicide Life Threat Behav 18:90–99, 1988.
39. Greenberg BS, Smith S, Yun JA, et al: The Content of Television Talk Shows: Topics, Guests and Interactions. Menlo Park, CA, Kaiser Family Foundation, 1995.
40. Grube J, Wallack L: Television beer advertising and drinking knowledge, beliefs, and intentions among schoolchildren. Am J Public Health 84:254–259, 1994.
41. Harris L and Associates: Sexual Material on American Network Television During the 1987–88 Season. New York, Planned Parenthood Federation of America, 1988.
42. Hazan AR, Lipton HL, Glantz SA: Popular films do not reflect current tobacco use. Am J Public Health 84:998–1000, 1994.

43. Heintz-Knowles KE: Sexual Activity on Daytime Soap Operas: A Content Analysis of Five Weeks of Television Programming. Menlo Park, CA, Kaiser Family Foundation, 1996.
44. Huesmann LR, Eron LD (eds): Television and the Aggressive Child: A Cross-national Comparison. Hillsdale, NJ, Lawrence Erlbaum, 1986.
45. Huesmann LR, Eron LD, Klein R, et al: Mitigating the imitation of aggressive behaviors by changing children's attitudes about media violence. J Pers Social Psychol 44:899–910, 1983.
46. Huesmann LR Eron LD, Lefkowitz MM, Walder LO: Stability of aggression over time and generations. Dev Psychol 20:1120–1134, 1984.
47. Huston AC, Donnerstein E, Fairchild H, et al: Big World, Small Screen: The Role of Television in American Society. Lincoln, NE, University of Nebraska Press, 1992.
48. Ile ML, Knoll LA: Tobacco advertising and the First Amendment. JAMA 264:1593–1594, 1990.
49. Jones EF, Forrest JD, Henshaw SK, et al: Unintended pregnancy, contraceptive practice, and family planning services in developed countries. Fam Plann Perspect 20:53–67, 1988.
50. Kalish DE (Associated Press): Hollywood can't seem to kick smoking habit. Albuquerque Journal, October 21, 1996, p D10.
51. Kunkel D, Cope KM, Colvin C: Sexual Messages on Family Hour Television: Content and Context. Menlo Park, CA, Kaiser Family Foundation, 1996.
52. Levine MP, Smolak L: Media as a context for the development of disordered eating. In Smolak L, Levine MP, Striegel-Moore R (eds): The Developmental Psychopathology of Eating Disorders. Mahwah, NJ, Lawrence Erlbaum, 1996, pp 235–257.
53. Levine MP, Smolak L, Hayden H: The relation of sociocultural factors to eating attitudes and behaviors among middle school girls. J Early Adolesc 14:471–490, 1994.
54. Madden PA, Grube JW: The frequency and nature of alcohol and tobacco advertising in televised sports, 1990 through 1992. Am J Public Health 84:297–299, 1994.
55. Malamuth NM: Pornography's impact on male adolescents. Adolesc Med State Art Rev 4:563–576, 1993.
56. Mediascope, Inc.: National Television Violence Study. Studio City, CA, Mediascope, 1996.
57. Mullin CR, Linz D: Desensitization and resensitization to violence against women: Effects of exposure to sexually violent films on judgments of domestic violence victims. J Pers Soc Psychol 69:449–459, 1995.
58. National Institute of Mental Health: Television and Behavior: Ten Years of Scientific Progress and Implications for the Eighties, Vol 1. Washington, D.C.: US Government Printing Office, 1982.
59. National Science Foundation: Research on the Effects of Television Advertising on Children: A Review of the Literature and Recommendations for Future Research. Washington, D.C., National Science Foundation, 1977.
60. Peterson RA, Kahn JR: Media preferences of sexually active teens. Presented at the annual meeting of the American Psychological Association, Toronto, August 26, 1984.
61. Peterson JL, Moore KA, Furstenberg FF Jr: Television viewing and early initiation of sexual intercourse: Is there a link? J Homosex 21:93–118, 1991.
62. Phillips DP, Carstensen LL: Clustering of teenage suicides after television news stories about suicide. N Engl J Med 315:685–689, 1986.
63. Phillips DP, Carstensen LL, Paight DJ: Effects of mass media news stories on suicide, with new evidence on the role of story content. In Pfeffer CR (ed): Suicide among Youth: Perspectives on Risk and Prevention. Washington, D.C., American Psychiatric Press, 1989, pp 101-116.
64. Princeton Survey Research Associates: The Kaiser Family Foundation Survey on Teens and Sex: What They Say Teens Today Need to Know, and Who They Listen to. Menlo Park, CA, Kaiser Family Foundation, 1996.
65. Shaffer D, Garland A, Gould M, et al: Preventing teenage suicide: A critical review. J Am Acad Child Psychiatry 27:675–687, 1988.
66. Shiffrin SH: Alcohol and cigarette advertising: A legal primer. Adolesc Med State Art Rev 4:623–634, 1993.
67. Signorielli N: Television and health: Images and impact. In Atkin C, Wallack L (eds): Mass Communication and Public Health. Newbury Park, CA, Sage, 1990, pp 96–113.
68. Singer JL, Singer DG, Rapaczynski W: Family patterns and television viewing as predictors of children's beliefs and aggression. J Communic 34:73–89, 1984.
69. Singer DG, Zuckerman DM, Singer JL: Helping elementary school children learn about TV. J Communic 30:84–93, 1980.
70. Strasburger VC: Adolescents, drugs and the media. Adolesc Med State Art Rev 4:391–416, 1993.
71. Strasburger VC: Children, adolescents, and the media: Five crucial issues. Adolesc Med State Art Rev 4:479–493, 1993.
72. Strasburger VC: Adolescents and the Media: Medical and Psychological Impact. Thousand Oaks, CA, Sage, 1995.

73. Strasburger VC: Children, adolescents, and television: An update. West J Med 166:353–354, 1997.
74. Strasburger VC, Brown RT: Adolescent Medicine: A Practical Guide. Philadelphia, J.B. Lippincott, 1997.
75. Strasburger VC, Furno-Lamude D: The effects of media consumption on adolescents' sexual attitudes and practices: Results of a pilot study [manuscript].
76. Strasburger VC, Hendren RL: Rock music and music videos. Pediatr Ann 24:97–103, 1995.
77. Surgeon General's Scientific Advisory Committee on Television and Social Behavior: Television and Growing Up: The Impact of Televised Violence. Washington, D.C., U.S. Government Printing Office, 1972.
78. Thomas K: No waiting to inhale: Cigarettes light up movies. USA Today, November 7, 1996, p D1.
79. U.S. Food and Drug Administration: Executive Summary: The Regulations Restricting the Sale and Distribution of Cigarettes and Smokeless Tobacco to Protect Children and Adolescents. Washington, D.C., FDA, August 23, 1996.
80. Williams TB (ed): The Impact of Television: A Natural Experiment in Three Communities. New York, Academic Press, 1986.

The Health Care Provider's Role in Adolescent Medical Decision-Making

M. MAX QUINN, J.D.
NANCY NEVELOFF DUBLER, L.L.B.

Division of Bioethics
Montefiore Medical Center
Bronx, New York

Reprint requests to:
Nancy N. Dubler, L.L.B.
Director, Division of Bioethics
Montefiore Medical Center
111 E. 210th Street
Bronx, NY 10467

This chapter presents three cases that illustrate the ethical issues that arise over decision-making in the health care of adolescents. The cases are then analyzed in the context of the set of principles and guidelines that grew out of an investigation into the ethical obligations of health care providers treating adolescents who are living without responsible adult supervision and guidance, referred to as the "adolescent alone."[4] We hope that this presentation not only demonstrates some of the issues present in treating such adolescents but also provides a framework for, and guidance in, thinking about how to resolve the issues that arise not only with adolescents alone, but with all adolescents.

CASE STUDIES

Case One: Refusal of Tracheostomy

AB was a very obese 17-year-old boy. His mother brought him to the hospital because she had become aware that he intermittently stopped breathing in his sleep. He was admitted to the hospital, and it was determined he was suffering from sleep apnea caused by his extreme obesity. It was believed that if he were to lose weight, the apnea would resolve. Weight loss would take some time, however, and the apnea was severe enough to be an immediate threat to his life. The doctors believed that the best course of action was a tracheostomy and that failure to perform this procedure would pose a serious risk to AB's life. AB, however, refused the tracheostomy. He did not discuss his reasons for refusing in great depth, but the impression he gave was that, because of previous frightening experiences with surgery, he was afraid of undergoing any surgical procedure. There was also some indication that he despaired of ever losing weight and had little motivation to try. He had been on several weight loss regimens in the past and none had succeeded. Because the doctors believed that his refusal put him at a serious risk of dying from the apnea, they tried many ways to convince him that this was the correct course of action. Discussions with physicians and nurses had emphasized the risk to his life, but caregivers were not sure that he fully understood the risk.

At first, the health care providers appeared to have two alternatives: (1) honor AB's wish for no surgery or (2) force the surgery over his objection. Choosing the first alternative would make the providers complicit in AB's risk of dying, and choosing the second would mean violating his physical person as well as vitiating his autonomy. Although no formal assessment of mental state had been made, AB seemed depressed. In addition, there was some reason to believe that he would agree to the tracheostomy if his fears about surgery in general could be addressed. In light of these concerns, the health care providers felt that simply acquiescing to AB's refusal and leaving him at a high risk of dying was ethically unacceptable. The risks of the surgical procedure for tracheostomy were few, and the risk of not performing the surgery was death. The health care team felt an obligation to respect AB's perspective, however, and they planned to do everything possible to allay his fears about the surgery and obtain his agreement to the tracheostomy. If all efforts of persuasion failed, however, the team felt that the risk of death was an unacceptable option. They also agreed that performing the tracheostomy and sending AB home with no support and no long-range, supervised plan for weight loss was equally unacceptable.

Because these alternatives were unacceptable, an attempt was made to arrange for continued hospitalization and implementation of a strict exercise and diet regimen until AB lost weight and no longer suffered from apnea, a plan that was expected to take at least 6 months. The team also requested psychiatric evaluation and support as a necessary part of AB's treatment for his obesity. Without this long-term plan in place for the boy's care, all agreed that performing the tracheostomy over his refusal, or even with his agreement, would be an inadequate and therefore ethically untenable plan.

Unfortunately, AB did not have any health care insurance, and his family could not afford to pay for the treatment. Appeals to the hospital to find some way to keep AB hospitalized failed. The adolescent unit had a limited supply of beds, and there was a concern that tying up one bed for so long would preclude treatment of children who needed more intensive medical care; although AB was going to need long-term supervision, he did not require complicated medication regimens. In light of this, the tracheostomy was not performed. After some searching, a rehabilitation facility was found that agreed to accept AB for long-term treatment of his obesity. He was transferred to the facility, but after a few weeks his disruptive and depressed behavior resulted in his being discharged from the facility.

Case Two: Noncompliance with a Medical Regimen for Severe Asthma Treatment

CD was a 17-year-old girl who had severe asthma most of her life. She had experienced more than 50 hospitalizations and in the 6 months prior to her latest hospital admission had been admitted to the ICU and intubated twice. She had an 8-month-old daughter and lived with her mother but spent weekends with the baby's father. Like most of her recent hospitalizations, the latest was the result of a severe asthma attack that had been brought on by her failure to take the appropriate medication on a regular basis. She had been prescribed an oral medication and a prescription inhalant, each of which she was supposed to use on a scheduled, rather than an as-needed, basis. She had used up her supply of medication and rather than calling or making an appointment to get more medication, she purchased an over-the-counter inhalant. The medical team responsible for her inpatient care agreed that for her severe asthma the over-the-counter medication was ineffective. In addition, because she hated being hospitalized, she would delay coming to the emergency room until she was almost completely unable to breathe. The medical staff felt that it was important for her to understand that treatment early in an impending crisis was crucial to avoiding prolonged hospitalizations, including possible intubation, and death.

As soon as CD's immediate crisis passed, she began to pester the house staff to discharge her. Engaging her in any conversation about her condition or treatment was difficult, because she seemed unable to focus on anything except getting discharged. Despite her age and single-mindedness, however, CD gave the impression of maturity. She complained that she could not take care of her daughter or even see her frequently while she was in the hospital. She also stated that she now felt as healthy as she ever felt. Medical staff realized that, although she had improved and the crisis had passed, she was not well enough to be discharged. In addition, they were certain that more asthma crises would ensue and CD might die unless some means of assuring her compliance with the required medication regimen were found.

Although CD was not articulating a refusal of treatment, her noncompliant behavior was sending a clear message. The health care providers responsible for her care were justifiably concerned both for CD's sake and for the sake of her daughter. Accordingly, they felt that the first step was to get her full attention, the next was to discover the barriers to her compliance with appropriate medication, and the final step was to overcome those barriers. A meeting was held in which many of those responsible for CD's care confronted her with their concerns. The providers were compassionate and understanding but made it clear to CD that she was risking her life and the well-being of her child. CD was surprisingly receptive and stated clearly that she did not want to die and leave her daughter without her mother. She also stated that she had no regular doctor and that getting refills for her prescriptions required a visit to a clinic. She often had to wait 4 or 5 hours before seeing a doctor, and she always saw someone who had never seen her before and who subjected her to a full examination and history-taking when all she wanted was her medication. She also avoided going to the clinic for medication because she was afraid that she would be hospitalized. CD said it was so much easier and "safer" to go to the drug store for an over-the-counter asthma inhaler.

The staff presented CD with several proposals. First, they made it clear, and CD understood, that her condition was too severe for an over-the-counter inhaler to be of any use. Next they proposed a bargain: a doctor would be found who could see her regularly to provide continuity of care and who would be willing to prescribe medications on the basis of a phone call, provided that CD agreed to visit that doctor at least once every 3 months for a check-up and comply with the medication regimen that was prescribed. In addition, CD agreed to come to the hospital as soon as she began to have difficulty breathing. An additional incentive was offered by the staff, who promised that they would do everything possible to discharge her within 24 hours and that they would be sensitive to her desire not to be hospitalized in the future but could not promise that she would never be an inpatient again. CD seemed relieved at the prospect of a regular doctor and also seemed to understand that if she kept her part of the bargain, she was not only less likely to require hospitalization but also greatly reduced her risk of dying. When asked whether she felt uncomfortable with any part of the plan, CD replied, "No, it's easy."

Case Three: Request for a Tubal Ligation*

EF was an 18-year-old woman with a 1-year-old child. She became involved with a man (not the father of her child) who infected her with HIV. Despite using condoms, EF became pregnant. Because of her religious convictions, EF would not consider aborting the child. She was nevertheless concerned about passing the HIV infection to the baby and about her responsibilities as a mother. She felt that bearing more children was irresponsible and morally wrong given the likelihood that she would die young and be unable to care for the children. Although she did not want to terminate the pregnancy, she felt it was important to ensure that she not become pregnant again. She therefore requested that a tubal ligation be performed immediately after the delivery.

While treating EF for her HIV infection, the treatment team developed much respect for her maturity and level of responsibility. In their discussions with her, it was clear that she had carefully thought through the consequences of her decision as well as the consequences of any further unwanted pregnancy. She was even asked how she would feel about having had the ligation if a cure for AIDS were discovered shortly after the ligation had been performed. Her reply was that she had to make her decisions with the medical facts as they currently exist: there is no cure. She could not risk the health of a future child or the likelihood of the child being orphaned at an early age because of a remote hope that a cure for AIDS will be found.

To consent for a tubal ligation in New York City, however, a woman must be 21 years of age, and EF therefore was not permitted under the law to consent to the procedure. The treatment team made many calls to lawyers asking them to help her get a court order permitting the procedure, but none was willing to accept her case. EF carried the baby to term and delivered. She and her health care providers continued to try to arrange for her to have the tubal ligation.

PRINCIPLES

The cases presented above illustrate a variety of ethical issues that arise in the context of the health care of adolescents. In a study that focused on the "adolescent alone," investigators identified four basic ethical principles that should govern a health care provider's approach to treating the adolescent patient: (1) respect for the adolescent's uniqueness and autonomy, (2) beneficence and nonmaleficence, (3) respect for the adolescent's need for support and guidance, and (4) justice.[4] The study also identified a set of guidelines that elucidate the principles. The guidelines are discussed below. Even though the "adolescent alone" investigation was particularly concerned with the ethical problems encountered in the health care of adolescents who are living without adult supervision, the principles and guidelines are applicable to the health care of all adolescents.

Respect for Uniqueness and Autonomy

The first principle states that the health care provider has a moral obligation to respect the adolescent as a unique person and to support the adolescent's developing autonomy. This principle should be recognizable as analogous to the well-established bioethical principle of respect for autonomy. In the context of the adolescent, however, the principle has been varied to take into account the developmental differences between adolescents and younger children on the one hand and adolescents and adults on the other. All children are engaged in the process of developing their own unique identities

*We are grateful to the health care team of the Montefiore Medical Center Adolescent AIDS program for sharing this case with us.

and becoming autonomous persons, but adolescents have reached the stage at which they need, want, and should be encouraged to exercise their skills in making the important decisions of their lives.[9,10] They have also reached the stage at which their basic cognitive skills are likely to be substantially similar to those of an adult, even though they lack the experience of adults in living and in decision-making. Moreover, they have a well-developed system of preferences and values. These may to some extent reflect the special pressures of adolescence, especially the need for peer approval, and if so, may evolve as the adolescent matures; nevertheless, they are the contemporaneous system by which the adolescent defines himself or herself and the foundation from which the more refined set of preferences and values will grow. If we accept that as adults we have general moral obligations to the younger generations, we must acknowledge that one of these moral obligations is to help them grow into the best adults they can be. We discharge this obligation with a combination of respect for their individuality and autonomy (just as we do an adult) and support in the face of their relative lack of experience and the evolving nature of their values and preferences. Respect for autonomy is assumed and generally honored unless it appears that such respect will cause undue harm to the patient.[5]

Each of the cases above raises issues about respect for the adolescent's autonomy. EF's case in particular demonstrates the importance of this principle. EF had a fatal disease and faced the prospect of leaving her two children without maternal care. In addition, she was very aware that she might transmit HIV to any other children she might bear. Despite her prognosis, she demonstrated an ability to think clearly about her future and that of her children. She did not distort the facts of her condition or the state of medical knowledge and ability to control HIV. EF demonstrated an extraordinary level of maturity and responsibility in the face of devastating life circumstances. Her efforts to make what would otherwise have been respected as a sound and responsible decision were thwarted by a rigid system that was established to protect youngsters, which in her case resulted in a violation of her rights.

CD's case appears to be about autonomy and choice, but a deeper probing reveals that it is really about a lack of access to care. CD appeared to be refusing care for her asthma but was actually responding to the lack of continuity and follow-up in her care. Her refusal resulted from her lack of humane, continuous, and thoughtful chronic care. In the evolving health care system, in which increasing numbers of poor adolescents will be parceled out to managed care plans or consigned to emergency rooms, discontinuous, episodic care is likely to alienate many patients and overwhelm their desire for care. As in CD's case, the barriers to care presented by a fragmented delivery system resulted in a "faux refusal," not an autonomous refusal that accepted the possible negative consequences.

Beneficence and Nonmaleficence

The second principle states that health care providers have a moral obligation to promote each adolescent's well-being and to minimize harm.[2] This principle again mirrors the general bioethical principles of beneficence and nonmaleficence. As stated above, some situations create a need to balance the principle of respect for the person and support for autonomy against potential harm from the exercise of that autonomy. An attempt to override a patient's autonomous choice is sometimes justified on the basis that acquiescence with the patient's wishes will cause unacceptable harm. In particular, when a disagreement arises between a provider and a patient, it is normally the case that the patient has made a decision and that the provider views the potential harm from that decision as unacceptable. The provider then finds himself or herself in a dilemma. He or she cannot strictly adhere to both the principle to support autonomy and the principle to minimize harm; a choice must be made. Most commonly the factor that resolves the dilemma is the patient's assessed decision-making capacity. Respect for and acquiescence to a patient's fully understood, fully considered decision that will result in harm or even death is generally considered the morally obligatory choice compared with forcing unwanted treatments. An even more complex dynamic is presented when caregivers consider withholding requested treatment, such as pain medication, because the caregiver has a misplaced fear that addiction will develop or the patient's life will be shortened. Disagreement with a fully understood, carefully considered decision made by a person having full decision-making capacity can be based only on a difference between the systems of values and preferences of the disagreeing parties. Our culture has a strong moral bias against forcing someone to live by the values of another. Therefore, the health care provider has a moral obligation to respect the patient's values, because these values are the result of patient deliberation and the frame of reality in which the patient exists and operates.

Because the health care provider is more than likely to have a different value system from that of the patient, the decision of a patient that is different from that which the provider believes he or she would make in the patient's position is not adequate evidence of a patient's lack of capacity to make the decision. It may be that the patient has deeply held values of which the provider is unaware or incapable of understanding fully because of cultural or personality differences. Therefore, a finding that a patient does not have the capacity to make a specific decision cannot be based on the choice that the patient has made in the circumstances, but must be based on criteria external to that decision, such as whether the patient fully understands the consequences of his or her decision and whether those consequences comport with a coherent set of values and preferences.

This analysis is important because the tendency to disregard a patient's choices because of a disparity in value systems is much greater when the patient is an adolescent. To some extent this is justified, since adults know from their own experience that values and preferences change between adolescence and adulthood, often quite dramatically. Many adults have regretted and suffered the consequences of decisions they made as adolescents that at the time were consistent with their values. As adults we hope to be able to guide and counsel adolescents and hope that they might benefit from our experience. This perspective, however, puts the respect for an adolescent's autonomy in greater jeopardy than respect for the autonomy of an adult. We see ourselves as wiser and we have more power in the social hierarchy; greater power must be wielded with enhanced care.

The case of AB raises the issue of a balance between respect for autonomy and avoidance of harm. Unquestioning respect for AB's autonomous choice to refuse a tracheostomy put AB at a serious risk of dying. Simply forcing the surgery on him was equally problematic. As discussed further below, the tension between respect for the adolescent's uniqueness and autonomy and the patient's well-being, which is often manifested by a patient's refusal of a treatment considered medically necessary, is a signal for deep, careful discussion between adolescent and caregivers.

In CD's case, allowing her to continue her noncompliant behavior without attempting to intervene also created a serious risk of death. CD's risky behavior, however, was not the product of a system of values and preferences that were incompatible with compliance with her medication regimen. Instead, access to adequate medical care was at the root of the issue.

Freedom from Abandonment of Aloneness

Unlike the first two principles, the third principle does not have an easy adult analogue among well-established bioethical principles, even though it is equally applicable to the socially isolated adult. The principle states that it is ethically unacceptable to require the adolescent to make decisions on his or her own without the possibility of consultation with a trusted adult. Because adolescents are almost but not fully adults, it is important that they have access to adult guidance and support. Even the most streetwise and grown-up teenager may need the wisdom and succor of a trusted adult. Sometimes the mere presence is sufficient, and the adolescent is able to make decisions on his or her own bolstered simply by the knowledge that the "net" is there if needed. In other cases, adolescents need adult consultation and advice. This need is unsurprising; few adults make weighty decisions without consulting their spouses, a trusted friend, or another significant person in their lives. Surely adolescents are no more independent than adults, although they may be pseudo-independent as a mask for fear. If a health care provider is aware that his or her adolescent patient is without such support, the provider should work to help the patient find a wise guide and companion.

In none of the cases presented was the need for a guide and companion specifically addressed, but it might have been appropriate in each case. Although AB's mother was involved, it is not clear whether she fulfilled the need for support for AB. It is often difficult for a parent to be a guide and companion to an adolescent child; however, in most cases it is all we have and, barring clearing indications of opposing interest, it is accepted and legally and ethically sufficient. In CD's case, a similar situation existed. Despite her noncompliance, CD presented herself as mature and had a child of her own. It was easy to overlook that she was herself in need of a companion and support that perhaps her mother and the father of her child were not providing. EF's case is similar in that she demonstrated such maturity that the need for support and guidance might easily have been overlooked. In addition, EF had a partner who might have been thought of as her support and companion.

Justice

The fourth principle is that a health care provider has a moral obligation to treat adolescents fairly, avoiding discrimination because of economic, social or familial circumstances, sexual orientation, race or ethnicity, or other personal characteristics.[2] In addition, the generally applicable principle of distributive justice is an issue for adolescents and adults. Although it is often not within the power of a single health care provider to distribute services fairly in an unfair and often unjust health care system, it is important to be alert to the fact that our health care system deprives many people of adequate care. Caregivers as advocates for their patients must struggle to overcome these systemic faults.

The cases of AB and CD clearly present issues of distributive justice. The absence of health insurance coverage restricted AB's access to the treatment he needed. Because no other means were available to compensate for this lack of insurance, it is possible, even likely, that AB will never be able to attain or maintain a healthy weight and will die much sooner than would otherwise be the case. Although it is not clear what behavior problems resulted in his discharge from the residential facility, it is possible that appropriate treatment for his psychological and emotional problems was not provided.

CD presents the classic situation in which socioeconomic status restricts access to health care. Unlike most of her middle-class counterparts, CD had no regular physician with whom she had established a relationship but instead needed to rely on overcrowded clinics and emergency rooms. In addition, she was caring for her own child, which made the hours spent waiting to get her medication even more burdensome. In CD's case, the outcome was more hopeful because the treatment plan involved connecting her with a physician who would agree to treat her on a regular basis.

EF's case presents a different type of justice issue. The law, created to protect women against coercive sterilization, discriminated against EF because of her age. This is a common problem with the law; there are many examples demonstrating the difficulty of writing law that is both general enough to protect those it is intended to protect and specific enough to allow for exceptions for the sake of justice or even common sense.

GUIDELINES

The "adolescent alone" project developed guidelines for health care professionals working with adolescents.[4] Many of the guidelines are implicit in the principles described above. The guidelines, discussed below, fall into four separate categories: (1) the adolescent's capacity and right to informed consent, (2) the adolescent's right to refuse and demand care, (3) the adolescent's right to confidentiality, and (4) the limits of the health care paradigm.

Capacity and Informed Consent

The guidelines define *capacity* as the ability to make an ethically valid decision on the basis of relevant information (such as the importance of the issue, personal values, and preferences) and to communicate the result of the decision-making process.[1] The guidelines stress that the notion of decision-specific capacity provides the appropriate context for a balancing of the principle of respect for autonomy and beneficence. In the case of an adolescent it is not enough to consider only the age of the adolescent; cognitive skills, moral development, life experiences, strengths and vulnerabilities, and current level of functioning all play a part in assessing an adolescent's decision-making ability.[4,6] With AB, for example, there was some reason to believe that he might lack the full capacity to refuse the recommended tracheostomy. He was possibly depressed and his fears about surgery and despair over ever being able to lose weight might have been affecting his ability to think clearly about the consequences of his refusal. CD, in contrast, clearly seemed to have full capacity but to be hampered by environmental factors in her motivation and ability to comply. EF's capacity to make the decision for tubal ligation as a matter of fact was unquestionable; her ability to carry out the ligation was precluded by the law.

It is important to pay careful attention to the adolescent's desire, or lack of desire, to make the decision for himself or herself—just as we would respect an adult patient's right to abdicate decision-making authority to a spouse, parent, or adult child if the patient felt too burdened by the disease and effects of treatments to make a decision. We recognize that disease and discomfort take a toll in physical and emotional energy and that a patient might technically have the capacity to make a decision but simply not have the energy or wherewithal. We should have the same respect for an adolescent and recognize that in some cases the emotional and physical reserves might even give out more quickly than in an adult. Some adolescents have had a wealth of experiences that have strengthened their decision-making skills, but others may be facing their first major life crisis and have no basis for having the confidence that they can make decisions. An adolescent who truly wishes to have his or her parents or other surrogate decision-maker take the leading role in treatment decisions has a right to have that wish respected.

Taking this last point to heart, however, requires the health care provider to assess carefully the adolescent's desires. This is not an easy task and must take into account not only current desires but the possibility that those desires might change rapidly. The task of orchestrating a balance between the adolescent's resources and his or her need for protection and care should not be underestimated.

A graduated decision-making model is incorporated into the guidelines. Under this model, as the potential for negative consequences increases, so should the concern about the adolescent's capacity. The cases of AB and CD illustrate this model. In both cases, the potential negative consequence was death. Accordingly, the initial refusal of each to agree to appropriate treatment to avoid the negative consequence was met with a great deal of concern on the part of the health care providers. Lengthy discussions among the providers and between the providers and the patients took place, and careful, sometimes agonized thought lay behind the ultimate decisions. A contrasting example might be an adolescent who is hospitalized with an uncomplicated broken limb and refuses daily needle sticks to monitor his or her blood counts. Honoring this refusal requires some consideration but not at the depth and intensity that the other examples require.

It is also important for health care providers to be aware of the legal environment in which they are operating.[8] A belief that the legal environment is harsher than it actually is and fear of legal repercussions might prompt caregiver to override the autonomous choice of an adolescent with full capacity. In contrast, a belief that the legal environment is more lenient might bring on lawsuits or unwanted legal reactions to actions that have overlooked a legal requirement.

Finally, when dealing with the issue of consent, the signature on the formal consent form may be that of the parent or other surrogate. It is important nevertheless to respect the adolescent's autonomy and engage in as full a discussion as possible with the adolescent about treatment risks and benefits and abide by the adolescent's decision. Difficult issues arise when parents and adolescents disagree about treatment. A full discussion of these issues is beyond the scope of this chapter. When parents and adolescents disagree over treatment, however, simply deferring to a parent's authority violates the mandate to respect the adolescent's autonomy. If the adolescent has the capacity to make the decision, the ethical requirement is to honor the adolescent's decision even when legal capacity is absent. Implementing this ethical requirement can place extraordinary demands on health care providers, who must at a minimum understand family dynamics and culture, the adolescent's developmental status, and the potential benefits and burdens of the decision in question.

The Right to Refuse or Demand Care

A refusal of care or a demand for care that a health care provider considers inappropriate or dangerous should be the beginning of a deep discussion with the adolescent and an attempt either to address the patient's concerns that give rise to the refusal or to find mutually acceptable alternatives to the recommended treatment. A refusal of recommended care always generates a health care provider's concern, and a refusal by an adolescent often elicits a strong paternalistic impulse as well. A demand for inappropriate or dangerous treatment elicits the same type of reaction. This impulse is appropriate, but the ethical response to it is not at either of the two extremes of simply abdicating on the one hand or forcing the provider's recommendation on the other hand. Instead, the health care provider's responsibility becomes that of engaging the adolescent in a discussion designed to determine whether there is a full understanding of the facts, whether developmentally appropriate concerns over things such as body image or peer judgments are in operation, or whether there are other potentially surmountable obstacles to the recommended treatment. If the factors motivating the adolescent can be addressed in a manner that satisfies the adolescent, consent will follow. If not, a process of determining a mutually acceptable alternative treatment should ensue.

The need for and use of this guideline is clearly demonstrated in each of the cases presented above. AB's refusal of treatment and CD's noncompliance should not have been, and were not, treated as the end of discussion of their care but the beginning of a series of discussions and negotiations over treatment. In both cases, health care providers demonstrated respect for the adolescent by taking the refusal or noncompliance seriously, but they did not simply capitulate in the face of the adolescent's apparent desire.

EF's decision had weighty and irreversible consequences and engendered a great deal of discussion with her health care providers, even though the treatment team respected her decision and believed that it was responsible and consistent with deeply held values.

Confidentiality

As with adult patients, health care providers have a moral obligation to respect and protect their adolescent patients' privacy and confidentiality.[3] Under certain circumstances, however, the health care provider has a contrary moral obligation to disclose facts about the patient (adult or adolescent), i.e., to breach confidentiality. Because of the special developmental significance of privacy to the adolescent, it is crucial that health care providers ensure that their adolescent patients clearly understand three basic elements regarding confidentiality: (1) absent a special circumstance, their discussions with the provider are strictly confidential and will be kept so; (2) the general nature of the special circumstances that require disclosure, such as suicidality, threat of harm to others, or a serious or chronic disease, such as cancer, requiring extensive and closely monitored care over a long time; and (3) if a circumstance requiring disclosure arises, the health care provider generally will not disclose any information without first discussing with the adolescent the nature of the information to be disclosed, the parties to whom it will be disclosed, and the reason that disclosure is necessary.

Limits of the Health Care Paradigm

The health care provider may play a more expanded role in the life of an adolescent than with an adult, and the inclination with adolescents, especially very needy adolescents, is to attempt to meet as many unmet needs as possible. It is important, however, for the provider to recognize and make clear to the patient the limitations of his or her role as provider, rather than as family, in the adolescent's life. Communication to the patient of the limits of the relationship is extremely important. This is not necessarily best accomplished by talking specifically about the limitations but rather by being clear in the interactions with the patient about where the boundaries are and what the provider can and cannot give to the patient. To be unclear about boundaries is to do a great disservice to the patient: expectations are created that certain of the adolescent's needs will be met by the provider, and the provider's failure to meet the expectations becomes one more disappointment to the adolescent.

CONCLUSION

In the process of maturing, adolescents walk a tightrope between childhood and adulthood; illness can threaten to upset their already precarious balance between the two stages in development. The health care provider also must walk a tightrope between helping to stabilize the balance and promoting, or at least hindering to the least extent possible, the process of becoming an adult. The principles and guidelines summarized above are intended to help health care providers to begin to capture the breadth and nuance of the circumstances that arise in the care of adolescents and to help them to maintain their balance.

References

1. Arras JD, Steinbock S: Ethical Issues in Modern Medicine, 4th ed. Mountain View, CA, Mayfield Publishing, 1995.
2. Beauchamp TL, Childress JF: Principles of Biomedical Ethics, 4th ed. New York, Oxford University Press, 1994.
3. Blustein J: Confidentiality and the adolescent: An ethical analysis. In Cassidy R, Fleischman A (eds): Pediatric Ethics: From Principles to Practice. Newtown Square, PA, Harwood Academic Publishers, 1996.
4. Blustein J, Levine C (eds): The Adolescent "Alone": Decision Making in Health Care, in press.
5. Brock DW: Children's competence for health care decisionmaking. In Kopelman L, Moskop J (eds): Children and Health Care: Moral and Social Issues. Norwell, MA, Kluwer Academic Publishers, 1989.
6. Buchanan AE, Brock DW: Deciding for Others: The Ethics of Surrogate Decision Making. New York, Cambridge University Press, 1989.
7. Dorn L, Susman E, Fletcher J: Informed consent in children and adolescents: Age, maturation and psychological state. J Adolesc Health 16:185–190, 1995.
8. Fleischman AR, Nolan K, Dubler NN, et al: Caring for gravely ill children. Pediatrics 94:433–439, 1994.
9. Holder AR: Legal Issues in Pediatric and Adolescent Medicine, 2nd ed. New Haven, CT, Yale University Press, 1985.
10. Moreno J: Treating the adolescent patient: An ethical analysis. J Adolesc Health Care 10:454–459, 1989.
11. Petersen AC, Leffert N: Developmental issues influencing guidelines for adolescent health research: A review. J Adolesc Health 17:298–305, 1995.

Confidentiality in an Age of Managed Care: Can It Exist?

CHARLES J. WIBBELSMAN, M.D.

Teenage Clinic
Kaiser Permanente Medical Center
San Francisco, California

Reprint requests to:
Charles J. Wibbelsman, M.D.
Chief, Teenage Clinic
Kaiser Permanente Medical Center
2350 Geary Blvd.
San Francisco, CA 94115-3305

Just as the pediatrician uses the otoscope as a basic tool in the examination of the child, so does the "ephebiatrician" use confidentiality as a basic tool in providing care to the adolescent. Confidentiality is the cornerstone of adolescent health care. Cheng et al. report: "Adolescent behavior, including care-seeking behavior, can be powerfully influenced by concerns about privacy."[4] For adolescents to know that they can be seen without a parent and that they can share what they may perceive as "unspeakable concerns" with a provider helps to break down traditional barriers for many teenagers. The rationale for this confidentiality is that adolescents engage in risk behaviors that require candid discussion with a health care provider. The American Academy of Pediatrics states that "adolescents tend to underutilize existing health care resources" and that lack of confidentiality is "a significant access barrier to health care.[17]

Adolescents seek medical care and medical advice in a variety of settings. They traditionally received care from the family physician in a fee-for-service model of health care delivery. Other models of health care, such as adolescent clinics in academic settings, were opened in the 1950s at Boston Children's Hospital in Boston and at Kaiser Permanente in San Francisco. These clinics provided adolescents with health care providers who had a special interest and training in caring for young adults and introduced adolescent medicine as a subspecialty in the United States.

Today, adolescents with confidential concerns who are unable to approach family members or the family doctor have sought out school counselors and other sources of health information. Many teenagers write letters to magazine or newspaper medical columnists. The *Dear Doctor* column in TEEN magazine often receives as many as 600 letters each month from troubled teens looking for help.[20] In an effort to seek confidential help, adolescents and young adults can now turn to the Internet and other sources of information without revealing their identity. Often, in an effort to preserve anonymity and safeguard their privacy, teenagers have simply signed their letters as "Worried in Wichita" or "Desperate in Denver."[14]

Today, with specific diagnoses required for reimbursement in some forms of managed care, the physician may function as an employee of an insurance carrier and thus may not be able to treat the adolescent confidentially. To guard the privacy of the adolescent, the physician may need to forgo the proper reimbursement. The challenge for health care providers of adolescents in managed care is to be able to deliver quality confidential care and not lose *control* of this care because insurance carriers require stringent reporting criteria.

CONFIDENTIALITY

This chapter analyzes the relationship between confidentiality and managed care. Readers also are referred to Adele Hofmann's discussion of ethical issues of confidentiality and consent.[8]

Consent laws vary from state to state. In states where parental notification or consent is required for a particular adolescent, health care issues such as termination of pregnancy,[1] ethical issues, and one-on-one bonding between provider and adolescent prevail and are critical. However, where the law does not require parental notification or consent, the mandates of confidentiality reign. A complete policy compendium of the consent laws of each state is available in a monograph from the American Medical Association entitled *Confidential Health Services for Adolescents*.[6]

Information regarding confidentiality is available from a number of other sources. The Society for Adolescent Medicine's *Position Paper on Access to Health Care for Adolescents* emphasizes confidentiality as one of several criteria for evaluating proposals to improve access to health care.[9] Strasburger et al. define statutory law, emancipated minors, the doctrine of the mature minor, emergency treatment, and confidentiality.[19] It is important for the health care provider to understand state consent laws and the legal rights of adolescents.

"Health care providers are in a unique position to establish a trusting relationship with adolescents and to confidentially explore these issues,"[3] states Cavanaugh. In summary, confidentiality is a vital part of quality care to an adolescent.

It is also critical to understand the differences between privacy and confidentiality. Patient privacy means that the health care provider respects the adolescent's dignity, as is shown by seeing the adolescent for a discussion and a physical examination without the parent or legal guardian being present. When a parent insists on being present in the examination room, the clinician may need to emphasize tactfully but firmly the importance of private time between the physician and the patient.

In another scenario, a provider may identify an issue protected by confidentiality in a visit such as a routine check-up of a 17-year-old girl who admits to being sexually active and requests contraception. The provider needs to respect the privacy of the adolescent and the dignity of the parent, who is often the health plan subscriber paying the premiums for care. Often the primary visit and interaction with the parent or guardian can be separate. The adolescent can be advised privately to return alone for a confidential visit to obtain contraceptives. Another frequent clinical scenario occurs when an adolescent, accompanied by a parent, is concerned about the possibility of being pregnant. A urine pregnancy test in the office setting can give the diagnosis without jeopardizing confidentiality that would be compromised by the use of a laboratory requisition or insurance coding.

Another major concern for many clinicians is breaking the bond of confidentiality between provider and adolescent. In a situation in which the well being of the adolescent is at stake—as might be the case with an adolescent who is suicidal or in crisis because of questions of sexual orientation—it is critical to include an adult with whom the adolescent is familiar, be it a parent, close friend, school counselor, or trusted teacher.

Finally, the age of the adolescent may be an important consideration. An 18-year-old seeking termination of pregnancy may be well served by the tenets of confidentiality. However, a sexually active, pregnant 12-year-old with the same request, even though protected in many states by the laws of confidentiality, probably would benefit from having the clinician's encouragement to include a trusted adult in the decision while the provider still maintains confidentiality.

It may be difficult to continue to provide confidential care in a managed care setting. In some instances, the best care may be via the county health department where confidentiality of care is not threatened by DRGs or insurance reporting. Often, the health care provider can be the facilitator for the transition between models of health care delivery.

MANAGED CARE

The traditional health care delivery system of fee for service is rapidly being replaced with different forms of managed care. All managed care is not the same. A private group model health maintenance organization (HMO) is not the same as a direct contract model HMO.

A newsletter published by the American Academy of Pediatrics in 1995 gives an excellent history and outline of managed care.[15] It points out that the three original managed care plan types were the managed fee-for-services, the preferred provider organizations (PPOs), and the HMOs, and it states that "managed care is a process of applying standard business practices to the delivery of health care in the tradition of the American free enterprise system."[15]

The traditional health care delivery system in the United States for the first half of the 20th century was fee-for-service care. For many, this was the only route to health care. For the adolescent, it meant there was only one choice: seeking medical care from the family physician, who would know the family and would send the parents a bill. In such a setting it was, and still is, difficult to ensure that confidentiality could be preserved and that the provider would be adequately compensated. The advantage of this type of health care is the familiarity of the adolescent and the family with the provider. The disadvantage is trying to protect confidentiality when collecting payment or simply not collecting payment for visits that require confidentiality.

Under the Federal HMO Act of 1973, an entity must have three characteristics to call itself an HMO: (1) an organized system for providing health care or otherwise assuring health care delivery in a geographic area, (2) an agreed upon set of basic and supplemental health maintenance and treatment services, and (3) a voluntarily enrolled group of people.[13] There are six common models of HMOs: the group practice model HMO and the staff model HMO, both of which are described below; the network model HMO, which is often a group of practices joined together that satisfy the criteria for an HMO; the IPA model HMO, in which the HMO contracts with an association of physicians to provide physician services to their members in return for a negotiated fee; the direct contract model HMO, in which the HMO contracts directly with individual physicians for services to HMO members; and the point-of-service model HMO, often referred to as an open-ended model, which allows health plan members to seek care outside of a specific network by having higher deductibles and copayments.[12]

Preferred provider organizations and the HMO models in which there is a *contract* between the HMO and the health care provider (as opposed to the group/staff model HMO) have the advantage that certain basic health care is paid for and included in the physician's provision of basic, comprehensive care to the adolescent.

However, disadvantages include that the provider is limited in reimbursement for a particular diagnosis and that the time spent with the patient may not be represented adequately in the reimbursement. Another disadvantage is that the contracts require a diagnosis for payment, and this may not permit keeping diagnoses confidential. There are model programs of managed care that can preserve confidentiality issues for the adolescent, offer basic health care in a comprehensive prepayment plan, and guarantee the adolescent quality preventive care in today's competitive health care industry's attempts to attract new members.

The Group and Staff Model HMO

The group model HMO such as the one at Kaiser Permanente is one model of managed care for adolescents. This health care delivery system allows health plan members, through a prepaid contract with the Kaiser Foundation Health Plan, to receive comprehensive and exclusive health care. This type of prepaid comprehensive care allows complete outpatient and inpatient care to adolescents with no or minimal copayments in a benefit package that ensures confidentiality. Many adolescents, realizing that they can receive comprehensive confidential care in a prepaid health plan, will use such services, particularly for contraception and screening for sexually transmitted diseases. Quality of care to adolescents and accessibility of services in a specific clinic for teenagers in a group model HMO such as Kaiser Permanente in Southern California has been documented by Klitzner.[10,11]

In a group model HMO, a private practice by a group of physicians (either a corporation or a partnership) contracts each year with a health plan (Kaiser Foundation Health Plan) to deliver specific services and benefits to health plan members exclusively. The advantage of this for the adolescent is that referrals are mostly within the medical group, which allows easier access to specialty services without jeopardizing confidentiality by needing to go outside the organization for medical authorization and care.

Staff model HMOs, such as Group Health Cooperative of Seattle or Harvard Pilgrim Community Health Care in Boston, differ from the group model in that the health care providers are employees of the health plan. However, the delivery of care and the "in house" involvement of the health care providers in the administration of the health plan is similar to the group model. This close involvement of the day-to-day "business" of the health care delivery system gives the provider much more control of his or her practice in the care of adolescent medicine. The disadvantages of the staff model HMO are that, as an employee of the health plan, the provider is under contract to the health plan in terms of compensation and benefits and is dependent on the strategic planning of the health plan's administration in matters that may require confidential care.

Many group/staff model HMOs have a history of providing structured care and confidential care to adolescents over the past 30 years.

In the 1970s there was only a fraction of the HMOs that exist today. Health care delivery for adolescents outside the traditional fee-for-service model was limited. In addition, if the adolescent did not belong to, or was unknowledgeable about, confidential prepaid services within the HMO, many teenagers needing confidentiality often sought out clinics administered by county health departments,[16] free clinics, Planned Parenthood clinics, or even mobile vans delivering health care to adolescents.[7] At that time, for health care providers wishing to practice quality adolescent medicine in a structured setting in which all services were available to adolescents under a single "umbrella of health care," the group or staff model HMO offered such an opportunity.

Group or staff model HMOs allow for the education of providers by specialists in adolescent medicine regarding confidentiality and consent issues. As pointed out by Fine, "Although HMOs currently offer some special services for adolescents, these are spotty and noninclusive."[5]

An established adolescent clinic in an HMO is a unique opportunity for providing confidential services to adolescents in managed care. Group model and staff model HMOs are uniquely suited to deliver this type of care.[10,11]

In San Francisco and Los Angeles, Kaiser Permanente has had free-standing teenage clinics for adolescents in a prepaid health system for more than 25 years. The success of these clinics stems from the existence of a separate place for adolescents to receive their medical care and the ability to provide adolescents with comprehensive one-stop confidential services. By being part of an established group model or staff model HMO, the teenage clinic easily gains referrals from other health care providers within the HMO and by marketing a health care delivery system just for adolescents. Not only is confidentiality the hallmark of these clinics, but having health care providers on staff who are interested and knowledgeable in adolescent health care issues contributes to the success.

An adolescent clinic within such an HMO model not only embraces confidentiality but, by offering adolescents easy access and no barriers to health care, can provide early intervention in medical crises and reap the benefits of preventive adolescent medicine and anticipatory guidance.

In 1982, there was one adolescent clinic in Northern California Kaiser Permanente, and the membership for the Northern California region was 1 million. Today the membership approaches 3 million members, and there are more than 10 teenage clinics. Similar growth has occurred at Kaiser Permanente in Southern California. As we approach the 21st century, this trend is expected to continue to provide quality, confidential medical care to adolescents.

CONCLUSION

This chapter has covered confidentiality and quality adolescent care as practiced in the group model HMO and the staff model HMO. We have seen that all managed care is not the same. Some forms of managed care, because of restrictive financial reimbursement of providers, severe limitations of referrals, and other forms of administrative restrictions on the practice of adolescent medicine, may compromise the confidentiality of medical care to adolescents. In such instances, the adolescent has little choice but to seek care outside the health care insurer.

References

1. Alan Guttmacher Institute: Teenage Pregnancy: The Problem Hasn't Gone Away. New York, AGI, 1981.
2. Brindis C, Wunsch B: Finding common ground: Developing linkages between school-linked/school-based health programs and managed care health plans. Sacramento, CA, 1996.
3. Cavanaugh RM: Obtaining a personal and confidential history from adolescents: An opportunity for prevention. Sexually Active Teenagers 1:34–38, 1987.

4. Cheng TL, Savageau JA, Sattler AL, DeWitt TG: Confidentiality in health care: A survey of knowledge, perceptions, and attitudes among high school students. JAMA 269:1404–1407, 1993.
5. Fine JS: The practice of adolescent medicine in staff model HMOs. HMO Pract 3:16–21, 1989.
6. Gans JE: Policy Compendium on Confidential Health Services for Adolescents. Chicago, Department of Adolescent Health, American Medical Association, 1993.
7. Guthrie AD Jr, Howell MC: Mobile medical care for alienated youths. J Pediatr 81:1025–1033, 1972.
8. Hofmann AD: A rational policy toward consent and confidentiality in adolescent health care. J Adolesc Health Care 1:9–17, 1980.
9. Klein JD, Slap GB, Elster AB, Schonberg SK: Access to health care for adolescents: A position paper of the Society for Adolescent Medicine. J Adolesc Health Care 13:162–170, 1992.
10. Klitzner IN: Meeting the challenge of adolescent health care in a group practice HMO. HMO Pract 7:151–156, 1993.
11. Klitzner IN, Borok GM, Neinstein L, MacKenzie R: Adolescent health care in a large multispecialty prepaid group practice: Who provides it and how well are they doing? West J Med 6:628–632, 1992.
12. Kongstvedt PR: The Managed Health Care Handbook, 3rd ed. Gaithersburg, MD, Aspen Publishers, 1993.
13. Managed Care Resource. Minnetonka, MN, United Health Care Corp., 1992.
14. McCoy K, Wibbelsman C: The New Teenage Body Book. Putnam, New York, 1992.
15. Merriman JT: The Beginner's Guide to Managed Care. The American Academy of Pediatric's Section on Adolescent Health Newsletter. Fall 1995.
16. Minkowski WL, Weiss RC, Lowther L, et al: Family planning services for adolescents and young adults. West J Med 120:116–123, 1974.
17. Policy Reference Guide: A Comprehensive Guide of American Academy of Pediatrics Policy Statements Published through December 1991. Elk Grove Village, IL, American Academy of Pediatrics, 1991, p 97.
18. Santelli J, Morreale M, Wigton A, Grason H: School health centers and primary care for adolescents: A review of the literature. J Adolesc Health Care 18:357–366, 1996.
19. Strasburger VC, Eisner JM, Tilson JQ, et al: Teenagers, physicians and the law in New England. J Adolesc Health Care 6:377–382, 1985.
20. Wibbelsman C: Questions asked in a Dear Doctor Column of TEEN magazine. Presented at the Annual Meeting of the Society for Adolescent Medicine, October 17–19, 1975, Washington, DC.

School-based Health Centers

PAMELA J. MURRAY, M.D., M.H.P.

Section of Adolescent Medicine
Department of Pediatrics
Children's Hospital of Pittsburgh
Pittsburgh, Pennsylvania

Reprint requests to:
Pamela J. Murray, M.D., M.H.P.
Director, Adolescent Medicine
Children's Hospital of Pittsburgh
3705 Fifth Avenue
Pittsburgh, PA 15213-2583

The number of school-based health centers (SBHCs) has rapidly increased over the past decade. In 1996, information about more than 900 comprehensive SBHCs was collected by Making the Grade of the Robert Wood Johnson Foundation. About 400 of these centers serve high school students. Comparable data from 1996 and previous years have been compiled annually by Advocates for Youth. The establishment of and, to a lesser degree, the ongoing presence of SBHCs have been controversial. The issue that dominated the early development was the explicit intent of some clinics to address reproductive health issues by offering contraceptive services. Subsequently, the possibility that other clinics might do the same, now or in the future, with or without sharing that intention, was the focus of controversy in many communities, even where reproductive health care was specifically excluded from the SBHC's array of clinical services. Some communities with high rates of HIV infection specifically advocated condom distribution. In other locales, where reducing the teen pregnancy rate was a priority, better access to effective hormonal contraceptives was the focus of controversy.

Once SBHCs are established, finances are most concerning to SBHC leadership. These issues are not as immediately controversial in the public arena, but attempts to resolve them have raised a new set of conundrums. Ongoing financial support must be found in state government and in the public and private health insurance sectors. Subsidies from foundations diminish as start-up phases evolve into maintenance financing. Managed care and capitated funding for primary health care have added new and problematic twists to the concerns about the financial viability and accountability of SBHCs.

Most of the first wave of SBHCs—those that offer the most experience and history—were established in high schools in the early 1980s.[15] In the growing number of middle and elementary schools with SBHCs, the clinical issues do not substantially change. However, the relative importance of parental involvement and concerns about the delivery of reproductive health care services assume greater significance.

Simultaneously, other influences on the health care system were gaining momentum. These included the emergence of the health care reform dialogue, a heightened debate about sexuality education, a focus on health services and outcomes research, and a move to privatize and decentralize public services. The advent of managed care and the unprecedented shifts in health insurance and the organization and ownership of health care institutions rapidly and radically changed the structure and practice of health care. Furthermore, the shift of Medicaid dollars to the state, the cutting back of reproductive health care funding, and ongoing organizational shifts in the health care industry continue to further threaten the health of adolescents. This is the context in which the controversies about school-based health centers must be considered.

SCHOOL HEALTH PROGRAMS

From the beginning of the 20th century, there has been an evolution of the role of health providers in the school setting.[14] The initial public health impetus was the control of infectious disease. Schools provided an opportunity for clinicians to reach young children in a relatively safe and reliable setting. Identification and treatment of infectious diseases set a precedent for screening for other conditions that could interfere with learning. Health initiatives with public health implications such as immunization tracking and campaigns continue to depend on the participation of school nurses. School nurses identify their professional role as providers, planners, and coordinators of students' health care. The mission of physical and health education in the curriculum also contributes to the spectrum of traditional comprehensive school-based health activity.

New Realities and New Opportunities

More recently, a flood of other resources addressing mental health and behavioral problems has flowed through schools.[21] These programs and providers often arrive in response to funding opportunities from government or private and foundation initiatives. Unfortunately, they often depart on a short fiscal timeline of government allocations or political interest. In the current era of collaboration, agencies requesting money often promise to deliver care at multiple sites. Schools are the best place to guarantee access to the greatest number of young people in need of almost any given service. As a result, many urban schools have large numbers of externally employed providers working on site. The school administration, inevitably trained and experienced in education but not in health or social service administration, has little direct authority over these guest providers. Space, supervision, and accountability are scattered. Unfamiliarity, short-term involvement, and limited opportunity to plan or evaluate globally or prospectively usually accompany this service patchwork.

Growing concerns about adolescent health and the lack of access to health care provided the stimuli for the establishment of SBHCs. The first SBHC was established in West Dallas, Texas, in 1970. This program attempted to provide comprehensive school-based health services at a high school to both pregnant and parenting adolescents.[19] Further attention was paid to the concept of school-based health services after the establishment of the now classic SBHC program in St. Paul, Minnesota. From the start, the goal of the St. Paul program was to reduce adolescent pregnancy rates, thus justifying the provision of reproductive health care within a comprehensive primary care model. The delivery of contraceptive services in this venue sparked both interest and opposition.

ADOLESCENT HEALTH PROBLEMS

Failing Health Status of America's Teens

Several reports issued in the 1980s highlighted the failing health status of America's teens.[7] The mortality rate of adolescents had not improved at the rate of other age groups since the 1950s.[10] Pediatric primary care maintained its emphasis on and commitment to anticipatory guidance and prevention, but American children were underimmunized, and teens were increasingly unfit and overweight. The Alan Guttmacher Institute's report on teen pregnancy highlighted national statistics about a rising pregnancy rate and the dramatic comparison to much lower rates in other industrialized countries.[1] The legalization of abortion and the broadened availability of effective contraceptives had not decreased the pregnancy and birth rates among unmarried teens. Educational and business sectors were concerned about the significant high school dropout rate and the poor academic skills of America's youth. Redefining the goals of adolescent health care and responding to its inadequacies became public health challenges with goals that were codified in Healthy People 2000 objectives.[10]

Adolescents visited physicians infrequently, and those that did usually only sought treatment of trauma and episodic illness rather than routine visits or preventive care.[7] Teens distributed their encounters among family practitioners, pediatricians, internists, obstetrician-gynecologists, allergists, and dermatologists. More providers were inviting adolescents into their primary care practices. Pediatricians were actively raising the age limits of their patients, internists were lowering theirs, and family practitioners were growing in numbers and distribution. Pediatric, adult, and family nurse practitioners and other midlevel professionals were establishing practices where adolescents were welcome, but adolescents still were not seeking comprehensive care. Patient-provider relationships did not have opportunities to develop and the lack of continuity of care mostly affected poor, urban populations.

New Morbidities and New Solutions

The new morbidities of the 1970s and early 1980s were summarized by the phrase "sex, drugs and rock 'n' roll." Recreational activities carried risks that included sexually transmitted diseases (STDs), pregnancy, drug abuse, and hearing loss. There were inescapable dangers and vulnerabilities in the day-to-day existence of teens living in urban, rural, and even suburban communities. Mental health problems in teens raised a parallel set of concerns. The adolescent suicide rate both increased and increasingly affected younger adolescents. The prevalence of violence generally and the homicide rate in particular were soon added to the agenda of adolescent health concerns.

The need for creative solutions for these concerns was endorsed by national leadership. For example, a statement by the American Medical Association in 1988 proposed a studied approach to the establishment of SBHCs and incidentally challenged the need to differently assess the outcomes of school health and primary care services.[7] Substantial support and funding came from foundations, most generously the Robert Wood Johnson Foundation. The Carnegie Foundation, the Federal Maternal and Child Health Bureau, and a number of state governments provided funding to support SBHC start-ups and evaluation. The Casey Foundation and local initiatives addressed some of the same concerns with a focus on educational and work readiness outcomes. Teen health issues were considered a treatable cause of truancy and a factor in the school dropout rate.

Teens who were uninsured, underinsured, and underserved by the distribution of health care resources had the greatest unmet needs. They experienced exceptional barriers to primary care, sometimes regardless of insurance status. Barriers of language and culture compromised the quality of care more frequently in impoverished communities. In the same poor neighborhoods, schools often had limited funds and resources for the traditional school health services. As was the case earlier in the century, schools were seen as the place to provide services to respond to problems that interfered with success at school.

In addition to the uninsured, underinsured, and underserved teens, pregnant and parenting teens were targeted as populations in need of, at least minimally, primary care services. They needed a broader scope of services that included pediatric and prenatal care, social support and coordination, and contraceptive services. Given the extraordinarily high rates of absenteeism and dropping-out among pregnant and parenting teens, an attempt to minimize barriers to health care and coordinate medical and social support was a logical plan of action.

Similarly, adolescents with chronic physical illnesses or significant psychiatric problems had specific health care needs and excess school absenteeism, and were thought to be able to benefit from school-based coordinated care and case management. In some chronic diseases, notably asthma and diabetes, frequent evaluation and education has been shown to improve disease management. Asthma, with its high prevalence among school youth and its enormous contribution to school absence, is a natural target for school-based intervention and outcome evaluation. Other diagnoses that make significant contributions to disability, morbidity, and school absence include other chronic medical and neuropsychiatric conditions, dysmenorrhea and other menstrual problems, STDs and associated conditions (vaginitis, urinary tract infections, pregnancy), upper respiratory infections, mood disorders, and other mental health problems.

An argument that has challenged SBHC advocates is that school-based services are not accessible to the highest risk youth, who are most likely to be truant, suspended, or dropouts. Others have argued that siblings, other family members, and recent graduates should not be excluded from using convenient school-based services. These concerns can have unique resolutions in each school and community. Enrollment or attendance may or may not be a requirement for use of a particular SBHC. Each SBHC may develop a mission statement and consequent policy guidelines that are based on need, resources, and accountabilities that will define the population able to use the SBHC. Failure to care for all the adolescents in a community is not a reason to neglect the needs of the majority. Most health problems and risks are sufficiently prevalent throughout the school-age adolescent population that opportunities for both prevention and intervention are legion.[8,13]

ROLE OF CONTROVERSY

Every SBHC has its stories of dissent and support. Opposition ranges from the rational to the extreme, and advocacy is found among anticipated and surprise sources. Individuals, community leadership, school boards, religious leaders, principals, parents, and youth contribute their opinions. Support of the school principal is the single most valuable, if not essential, element. Leadership of the sponsoring agency must believe in the concept and work for the SBHC's establishment. As with many issues, supporters are generally less organized and outspoken than the dissenters. Religious and other community leaders who support the provision of health services to the underserved exist in every community and should be contacted and encouraged to verbalize their support. Opposition most often influences the range of services that are approved by the host authority. Planning committees should be prepared to respond to the content and tactics of organized opposition. People who speak in public forums often benefit by some rehearsal or training in dealing with disruptive opponents who may challenge the normal rules of order.

Rienzo reports on this aspect of SBHC development by reviewing and evaluating five case studies.[17] An awareness of the scope and magnitude of identified health and community problems is necessary for recruiting support. Providing a needs assessment and quantitative data to support the SBHC helps to engage advocates and communicate the need to a wider audience. Key players who have the ability to communicate a plan that appears to be fundable and realistic and the ability to show potential benefits of the SBHC's success further the cause. Objective surveys of students, parents, and teachers have demonstrated overwhelming support, particularly when the specific policies of and the limits to reproductive health care are explicitly stated. In addition to the original needs assessment, polls can be persuasive to school administrators and boards. Positive media attention can promulgate facts about health care needs and the SBHC's plans to a larger community and catalyze support on an informed basis.

REPRODUCTIVE HEALTH AND SEXUALITY ISSUES

Sexuality issues dominate the debates on reproductive health education, but this is not unique to SBHCs. These issues are similarly debated in forums in varied contexts and settings discussing sex education, abortion, family planning, and minors' rights to access reproductive health care. A broad range of reproductive health services, including the evaluation and treatment of STDs; the counseling, prescription, and dispensing of birth control; the distribution of condoms for any reason; and the diagnosis of pregnancy, the communication of pregnancy options, and pre- and postnatal care have been proposed at various SBHCs. The resolution of these issues and ultimate provision of services varies among sites. Issues of consent and confidentiality are also generic to the broader scope of adolescent health care regardless of the site of delivery. The legal framework is a three-dimensional patchwork of federal, state, and local guidelines codified by courts, legislation, and regulations, and they are often left open to interpretation and challenge.

Provision and Utilization of Services in Schools

Full-service SBHCs, across the board, report that 10–20% of visits in high schools are for reproductive health care.[16] Peak and Hauser-McKinney summarize the availability and range of reproductive health services offered at 180 school-based or school-linked health centers from a 1993 survey.[16] Overall, 20% of visits were for reproductive health concerns; 109 of the responses were from school-based programs. Most sites provided some reproductive health services. In the SBHCs, counseling, follow-up of contraceptive use, gynecologic exams, and pregnancy counseling options were available at most SBHCs. About a third of the SBHCs provided prescriptions for contraceptives, condoms, and diaphragm fitting. About 15% distributed oral contraceptives and foam; and 1% made available long-acting progestogen contraceptives. Notably, most of the SBHCs that provided contraceptives and condoms had done so since they opened. Condoms were more likely to be added at a later date, which may reflect growing concerns about HIV infection in the adolescent population more than an expansion of family planning methods. The SBHCs in existence the longest, 10 years or more, were the most likely to dispense contraceptives and condoms. These centers, which were established in the early 1980s, were likely to have been influenced by novel approaches to decreasing the teen pregnancy rate.[9] This counters the perception that SBHCs insidiously introduce birth control into the school setting.

About 90% of school districts impose some restrictions on service delivery.[16] In five of six SBHCs, a restriction on the provision of contraceptive services was identified.

Additional restrictions were dictated by state policy, the sponsoring agency, and health center policy in only a few centers. Although centers providing reproductive health services and contraception cite high utilization of these services, an impact on individual or community health outcomes is still unproven. From our observations of adolescents' difficulties with contraceptive-seeking behavior, appointment-keeping behavior, and compliance with contraceptive choices, we expect that the proximity of services and the relative ease of follow-up could enhance effective use of pregnancy and STD prevention options for some individuals. Nonetheless, comprehensive SBHCs alone have not been able to document reductions in community teen pregnancy rates.[13,19]

Perinatal Care

A case control study of pregnant and parenting teens in West Dallas, Texas, focuses on adolescents committed to continue their pregnancies.[19] Comprehensive school-based services increased the number of prenatal visits. Maternal pregnancy complications were less common in the SBHC group, but neonatal outcomes of gestational age and birthweight did not differ. School enrollment was higher during and immediately after the pregnancy in the SBHC attendees, but school dropout rate and repeat births converged in the two groups in the first and second postpartum year, respectively. Other comprehensive programs for pregnant and parenting teens have similarly demonstrated a limited ability to decrease repeat pregnancy rates for just the 12 months following delivery. When the care in the comparison group had similar goals and organization, the outcomes were similar. This reinforces the importance of broader social and cultural influences on the problem of teen pregnancy and its consequences. Perhaps certain program attributes may contribute to specific outcomes. Further analyses may reveal lower costs for similar outcomes when prenatal care is provided in the school setting. This may allow for enhanced provision of additional services that address some of the persistent school retention and repeat pregnancy problems.

EDUCATION–HEALTH CARE INTERFACE

Some critics have stated that schools should only teach and not become involved with other issues of child health and welfare. However, with funding sources emphasizing interagency collaboration, many youth-serving agencies try to collaborate with and place their staff in schools. The advantages associated with the service delivery are similar to those offered by SBHCs; they minimize barriers to access and are expected to improve appointment-keeping compliance.[13] Because these services are often problem-focused and staffed only part-time at any one site, they may never have the opportunity to integrate with the school community. They pose administrative and logistic challenges and operate as satellites of the parent agency. There is a lack of time to meet or collaborate with other school-based services. Larger schools commonly have dozens of independent outside agencies contributing some human resources to the school. SBHCs, because of their controversial visibility, intense development phase, parental consent requirement, and frequent need to work with the school on resolving day-to-day issues, are often less alien to the school culture, administration, and community.

Confidentiality

In the SBHC, as in other institutional settings of a nonmedical nature, careful definition of confidentiality guidelines is advised. Administrators of schools and the sponsoring agencies, students, parents, and other staff have expressed concerns about the confidentiality of SBHC encounters. Specifically, policies and procedures concerning mental health diagnoses and care, drug evaluations and treatment, HIV testing and status, and other communicable diseases including STDs justify definition and clarification. The patient-specific issues are generic for the delivery of adolescent health care, and there is potential for conflict among patient, parents, and practitioners. The patient's record is treated like any other medical record and never as school property.

A study by Cheng surveyed students in three Massachusetts high schools about confidentiality issues.[4] Only a third of students demonstrated an awareness of rights to confidential care. More than half claimed to have health concerns that they wished to keep from their parents; even more wished to keep those concerns from their friends and classmates. Whereas almost all students with a regular source of care would visit their physician for a physical illness, only slightly more than half would go to that physician for a sensitive issue, such as pregnancy, AIDS, or substance abuse, that they wished to keep private. Yet the regular physician still ranked higher than any of the other choices in the perceived assessment of privacy and the adolescents' willingness to use that source of care. Students who had previously used the SBHC or who had discussed privacy issues in a health care setting had better opinions of confidentiality than those who had not. While this demonstrates some positive outcomes from SBHC use, the lack of knowledge about rights to confidential care, reluctance to use regular and available care for private issues, and the highlighted concerns about the confidentiality available in a SBHC raise many questions about perceptions of confidentiality and its actual influence on health-seeking behavior.

Mental Health Services

Issues of scope, financing, integration, and confidentiality are critical to the planning and implementation of mental health services of adolescents. The experience of the early SBHCs confirmed the need for psychosocial services for adolescents who used the SBHCs. Medical providers were often overwhelmed by the demand and professionally unprepared to provide the needed evaluation and interventions. The supply of mental health providers was insufficient to meet the identified needs. Both in collaboration with and independent of SBHCs, new models for the delivery of mental health services to adolescents in the school setting have been pioneered.[21]

Training

Training opportunities in a school-based setting may influence subsequent practice styles and choices.[11] Future interest and participation in school health issues is influenced by exposure as a trainee.[5] Participation in a school's or SBHC's activities allows trainees to observe normative behavior of adolescents and to interact with adolescents in their everyday environment. A firsthand awareness of peer interactions can be as enlightening as seeing the same adolescent with and without a parent present.

Research

Academic investigation poses unique challenges and opportunities. Smaller-scale projects are within the scope of many SBHCs. The school principal may be an excellent sounding board and needs to know of any plans before they are discussed or presented at any school or public forum. School boards and school district institutional review boards (IRBs) may have different priorities than academic IRBs. Concerns about confidentiality of the school and the school district, in addition to that of the student, may be a major concern. The discussion of "sensitive" topics, regardless of the benefits or outcomes, may pose political problems for the school and consequently for the SBHC.

COMPETITION

Initially there was little opposition to SBHCs from individual physicians. As SBHCs become more widespread, establish themselves in middle or mixed income communities and schools, and compete for fewer and more restricted health care dollars, medical opposition may become more visible. Medical practitioners may object to the potential reorganization of care patterns and question the quality or necessity of school-based health care visits. States that have not resolved issues related to the roles and scope of midlevel providers may see SBHCs as another battlefield for interprofessional conflict. Alternatively, cost-benefit and outcome studies of pediatric primary care practice may encourage pediatricians to care for more complex problems, with midlevel practitioners providing increasing amounts of well-child and minor illness care. Saving parents and adolescents the indirect costs of health care (time off work and school, waiting times, transportation and parking costs) may be attractive to segments of the population, particularly single and working parents from a variety of socioeconomic backgrounds. The current health care market's enhanced economic awareness and concern with patient satisfaction could promote some advantages of SBHCs compared with, or in combination with, other sites.

The SBHC setting is recognized as an opportunity to establish confidential and supportive relationships between providers and patients. It succeeds in providing services to underserved adolescents, but there is lack of evidence supporting their ability to alter behaviors or improve health outcomes. The American Academy of Pediatrics' Committee on School Health and other advocates of comprehensive school health recommend that SBHCs attempt to strengthen behavioral change outcomes by targeting students most at risk and engaging in more outreach in the school and the community. The challenges to SBHCs are valid but apply similarly to the broader practice of adolescent primary care.[18]

MANAGED CARE

The focus of public debate and the literature has shifted to issues related to managed care.[2,3,23] This concept has unified the concerns of insured patients regardless of the source of their insurance and thus affects most potential SBHC users. Insurers are more likely to insure members of both privately and publicly funded plans. Coverage in both sectors is more often capitated, particularly for primary care. Additionally, the trend is for governments to remove themselves from direct provision of or payment for health services and instead to contract for or privatize needed services. Programs directly funded by the government are threatened if state governments are already contracting and paying another entity to "cover lives"—regardless of whether the patient goes for appointments, some health care provider is receiving funds for that patient's primary care and care management. If SBHCs are to survive, they need to create formal relationships with managed care organizations. Three variations are commonly proposed: independent, complementary, and collaborative relationships.

If SBHCs can meet the service and availability requirements for a primary care provider (PCP), their staff may become designated PCPs in one or more managed care plans. This is an option for some SBHCs linked to larger institutional networks of hospitals and community clinics and practices where the SBHC and affiliated providers **independently** provide all primary care. In markets where PCPs are expected to work exclusively within one network, a link to one managed care program may exclude students in another program from using the SBHC's services. Without external regulation, a decision to align with a plan that demands exclusivity could undermine the philosophic core and initial rationale for the establishment of SBHCs.

The second organizational relationship is a **complementary approach** that creates a specialist status for the SBHC's providers that requires referral from a PCP for reimbursement. Exceptions to the referral requirement might include mental health, family planning, and other preauthorized services. PCP approval is likely to be limited to inexpensive services that improve other plan performance measures, such as immunizations. These services would not justify the quantity and skill of most SBHCs' staff and would be more fitting in situations in which the only staff is the school nurse, a model that some school districts are moving toward independently.

The third and last model proposed is a **collaborative primary care model**, where capitated funds, ideally from multiple plans, support the SBHC. Communication between collaborative sites is critical. Electronic medical records and facsimile machines reduce the delay and work of sharing medical information between identified sites. The SBHC can facilitate the provision of some sensitive or confidential services. It also has other applications, including the provision of health care to older adolescents attending college away from home; such an explicitly shared model avoids emergency visits, fragmented care, and medical neglect when the patient is living away from the PCP's site.

There can be significant administrative costs to join managed care arrangements. If sponsoring agencies can include SBHCs in their larger-scale negotiations, the SBHC staff will be spared from some uncertainties and responsibilities. Instead, they can inform the network of their plans and needs for communication and database infrastructure and invest time in developing relationships with their primary care partners, as they did with their school health colleagues.

THE FUTURE

The current focus on parents' rights and self-determination in education, the increase in home-schooling, the lack of national health insurance or progressive health reform, and the current decentralization and dismantling of federal social welfare programs all speak to the political atmosphere of this time. The safety net in our communities and the concerns for the health and welfare of the underserved are not high on the political agenda.

The emphasis on profit, and the shift of control to the insurers from hospitals and physicians, is sending waves of change across the health care industry. SBHCs are a small item in the overall cost scheme. They can be easily eliminated or forgotten; they can also be used for promotion and image. Who will negotiate for and about the health centers is critical. To survive, they will need vertical integration with sponsors and networks and the support of users, schools, and parents. They also will need horizontal integration on a geographic scheme to negotiate with governmental departments that fund public health services.

What might have been presented as one more point of controversial interest has rapidly evolved into a challenge for survival for many SBHCs. Changes in health care financing for the publicly insured are undermining the program block funding and fee-for-service reimbursements that contribute more than 50% of current SBHC revenue. Some communities are looking to the once less accessible mental, and even dental, health services that are "carved out" of managed care plans to provide some financial infrastructure for SBHCs. But inevitably SBHCs must find a way to negotiate, collaborate, and contract with managed care entities to survive. They will also need support from purchasers of health care and voters, the parents of students and students themselves, and education and health care professionals. The latter groups are experienced at advocacy but are consumed with crises of major systemic challenge in private and public sectors. Neither public education nor private health insurance, once stable elements of their larger system, may be the same by the end of this decade. School-based health centers, dependent on and influenced by these institutions, are viable and vulnerable. A rational look at adolescent health problems continues to support thoughtful and evaluated approaches to prevention and intervention. School-based and community-linked services provide promising opportunities[8,13,22] to demonstrate effectiveness by integrating primary care and public health activities, critical elements associated with improved community and individual health status measures.[18,20]

References

1. Alan Guttmacher Institute: Teenage Pregnancy: The Problem Hasn't Gone Away. New York, AGI, 1981.
2. Brellochs C, Zimmerman D, Zink T, et al: A partnership for quality and access: School-based health centers and health plans, school health policy initiative. Washington, DC, Janin/Cliff Design, 1996.
3. Brellochs C, Zimmerman D, Zink T, English A: School-based primary care in a managed care environment: Options and issues. Adolesc Med State Art Rev 7:197–206, 1996.
4. Cheng TL, Savageau JA, Sattler AL, DeWitt TG: Confidentiality in health care: A survey of knowledge, perceptions and attitudes among high school students. JAMA 269:1404–1407, 1993.
5. Chilton LA: School health experiences before and after completion of pediatric training. Pediatrics 63:565–568, 1979.
6. Committee on School Health, Nader PR (ed): School Health: Policy and Practice. Elk Grove Village, IL, American Academy of Pediatrics, 1993.
7. Council on Scientific Affairs: Providing medical services through school-based health programs. JAMA 261:1939–1942, 1989.
8. Dryfoos JG, Klerman LV: School-based clinics: Their role in helping students meeting the 1990 objectives. Health Educ Q 15:71–80, 1988.
9. Edwards LE, Steinman ME, Arnold KA, et al: Adolescent pregnancy prevention services in high school clinics. Fam Plann Perspect 12:6, 11–14, 1980.
10. Healthy People 2000: National Health Promotion and Disease Prevention Objectives. US Public Health Services, Department of Health and Human Services, Washington, DC, US Government Printing Office, 1991.
11. Juszczak L, Fisher M, Lear JG, et al: Training opportunities in school-based health centers. Dev Behav Pediatr 16:101–104, 1995.
12. Kirby D, Resnick MD, Downes B, et al: The effects of school-based health clinics in St. Paul upon school-wide birth rates. Fam Plann Perspect 25:12–16, 1993.
13. Kirby D: Comprehensive school health and the larger community: Issues and a possible scenario. J Sch Health 60:170–177, 1990.
14. Lear JG: School-based services and adolescent health: Past, present, and future. Adolesc Med State Art Rev 7:163–180, 1996.
15. Lear JG, Gleicher HB, St. Germane A, et al: Reorganizing health care for adolescents: The experience of the school-based adolescent health care program. J Adolesc Health 12:450–458, 1991.
16. Peak GL, Hauser-McKinney DL: Reproductive and sexual health at the school-based/school-linked health center: An analysis of services provided by 180 clinics. J Adolesc Health 19:276–281, 1996.
17. Rienzo BA, Button JW: The politics of school-based clinics: A community-level analysis. J Sch Health 63:266–272, 1993.
18. Santelli J, Morreale M, Wigton A, Grason H: School health centers and primary care for adolescents: A review of the literature. J Adolesc Health 18:357–366, 1996.
19. Setzer JR, Smith DP: Comprehensive school-based services for pregnant and parenting adolescents in West Dallas, Texas. J Sch Health 62:97–102, 1992.
20. Starfield B: Public health and primary care: A framework for proposed linkages. Am J Public Health 86:1365–1369, 1996.
21. Taylor L, Adelman HS: Mental health in the schools: Promising directions for practice. Adolesc Med State Art Rev 7:303–317, 1996.
22. Vincent ML, Clearie AF, Schluchter MD: Reducing adolescent pregnancy through school and community-based education. JAMA 257:3382–3386, 1987.
23. Zimmerman DJ, Reif CJ: School-based health centers and managed care health plans: Partners in primary care. J Public Health Manage Pract 1:33–39, 1995.

Should Adolescents Have Over-the-Counter Access to Oral Contraceptive Pills and Antibiotics?

GERI D. HEWITT, M.D.

Clinical Assistant Professor of Obstetrics and Gynecology and Pediatrics
Ohio State University College of Medicine
and
Ohio State University Medical Center and Columbus Children's Hospital
Columbus, Ohio

Reprint requests to:
Geri D. Hewitt, M.D.
4053 Dublin Granville Rd.
Dublin, OH 43017

The United States has the highest rates of teenage pregnancy and abortion in the industrialized world. Few would argue that these rates are unacceptably high; the controversy centers on the best solutions for this problem. Approximately one-half of American adolescents become sexually active by the age of 17 years,[2] and most adolescents delay seeking medical care for contraceptive services for an average of 1 year after the onset of sexual activity.[17] Yet one-half of all adolescent pregnancies occur in the first 6 months of sexual activity when most adolescents have not sought medical care for contraceptive services.[17] Approximately 41% of 15–19-year-old girls used no form of contraception at their first sexual encounter.[15] Adolescents under the age of 15 years are particularly at risk for pregnancy during this period.

Oral contraceptive pills (OCPs) are an effective form of contraception with few contraindications in healthy adolescents.[13] Some argue that by eliminating the mandatory requirement of interaction with a health care provider before initiating OCPs, patients will have more direct access and be more likely to use them. Should healthy adolescents be able to obtain OCPs that provide effective contraception with minimal if any risk without first interacting with a health care provider? Would eliminating this interaction increase the proportion of sexually active teenage girls using hormonal contraception, particularly when they first become sexually active?

How does the sexually active adolescent benefit from interacting with a clinician before initiating

OCPs? Are the potential benefits great enough to justify delaying the initiation of OCPs until after such an interaction takes place? Is this interaction a significant barrier that needs to be eliminated to increase the percentage of sexually active adolescents who are successful contraceptors? Would over-the-counter availability of other relatively safe medications commonly used by sexually active girls, such as antibiotics to treat vaginitis or sexually transmitted diseases (STDs), decrease the incidence of untreated STDs and their sequelae, such as pelvic inflammatory disease, infertility, ectopic pregnancy, and chronic pelvic pain? Would we improve the overall emotional, mental, and physical health of adolescents by eliminating the barrier of interaction with a health care provider to obtain such medications? I argue that interaction with a health care provider before initiating medications such as OCPs or antibiotics for an STD is crucial in the overall health of adolescents. One hopes that clinicians provide adolescents with much more than just a Papanicolaou smear, pelvic exam, and renewal of birth control pills during these encounters.

BARRIERS TO GYNECOLOGIC CARE AND CONTRACEPTIVE SERVICES

What are the barriers to health care, specifically gynecologic care and contraceptive services, that adolescents face? Would making medications available over the counter eliminate these barriers? What other methods may be more effective in removing these barriers?

Lack of financial resources to pay for outpatient visits, laboratory fees, and prescription medications is a potential problem for adolescents of all economic backgrounds. Even if covered by private medical insurance, some adolescents are unable or unwilling to use their insurance because of concerns about parental notification and consent. Even if they are able to use their parents' health insurance, not all policies cover preventive health care and contraception. Concern about parental discovery is an important issue for adolescents who fear parental discovery and its perceived or real negative ramifications if they seek contraceptive services. Even if they are able to confide in their parents, some girls still may not have access to the necessary financial resources, and few adolescents have the cash available to pay for such services or lack the resources to find confidential, affordable care. Most adolescents report that maintaining confidentiality and making contraceptives easy to obtain at no cost would improve contraceptive use and compliance.[11] Many of these financial restraints would not be eliminated unless making OCPs available over the counter was accompanied by a drastic reduction in cost.

What barriers other than financial constraints keep sexually active adolescents away from our offices and clinics, even though they need gynecologic and contraceptive care? Fear of undergoing a pelvic examination is cited by patients who have never had an examination as well as patients who have had several examinations as another reason to avoid or delay interaction with a health care provider. Yet studies have shown that delaying the pelvic exam for up to 6 months after the onset of use of hormonal contraception has no negative effect on the patient's health.[5] Perhaps selectively delaying the pelvic exam in asymptomatic and otherwise healthy girls until a rapport has been established between patient and clinician would improve the experience for the patient and make it less feared.

Lack of transportation to clinics is a problem for some adolescents as well as finding clinics that provide care during times compatible with school and work schedules. Clinics need to be placed close to and preferably within walking distance of where adolescents live, work, and go to school and need to be open at times when adolescents are able to benefit from their services.

Many adolescents have difficulty with finding clinics that provide age-specific, culturally sensitive care by a knowledgeable and attentive staff. Once a patient makes her way to a clinician, expresses her need for contraception, and undergoes an examination, she may or may not be given the contraception that she is seeking. One poll showed that only 32% of pediatricians would prescribe OCPs for a 15-year-old adolescent seeking contraception, and only 35% would consider doing so without parental consent. Adolescents seeking contraceptive services from obstetricians and gynecologists fare better; 92% of obstetricians and gynecologists report that they would prescribe OCPs to a similar patient, with 18% requiring parental consent. Of even greater concern is the fact that only 61% of the pediatricians polled would refer the patient to a clinician who would provide them with confidential contraceptive services.[14] Clearly not all clinicians feel comfortable dealing with the issues of adolescent sexuality and need for contraception. Education may allow these clinicians to feel more comfortable with providing such services to all adolescents or at least lead to an appropriate referral to a clinician who can meet the patient's medical needs. Physician prescribing practices and lack of referral to an appropriate clinician should not be barriers to obtaining safe and effective contraception.

PATIENT EDUCATION AND COUNSELING

Educating adolescents about issues pertaining to sexuality and contraception has many important ramifications. Scandinavian countries have a similar rate of teenage sexual activity but a much lower rate of teenage pregnancy. One reason postulated for this difference is the early and universal sex education programs in school.[15] American adolescents also have been shown to benefit from sex education. They show more accepting attitudes about their own and others' sexuality, and they are more likely to use contraception at their first sexual encounter if they have received formal education about issues pertaining to sexuality and contraception.[12] Adolescents who undergo sex education are no more likely to initiate sexual activity than those who are uninformed.[12]

Access to information about sexuality and contraception is more limited in the United States than in other countries.[15] The sources available to adolescents to gain such information include parents, friends, siblings, partners, religious or community programs, health care providers, and school. Certainly some of the sources are more reliable and informative than others. Studies have shown that contraceptive behavior is influenced by the media, public opinion, and attitudes of health care providers.[15] One study found that, when asked, 66% of adolescents would like to discuss contraception and 70% would like to discuss STDs with their doctor. Unfortunately, only one in five adolescents had actually discussed these issues with a clinician.[11]

With limited access to sound information about sexuality and contraceptives, it seems foolish to eliminate a potentially positive interaction with clinicians. Discussion with health care providers also can help with the adolescent's self-esteem, decision-making skills, and communication skills. Health care providers also can encourage or facilitate parental disclosure about the adolescent's sexual behavior. Some studies suggest that parental involvement increases the effectiveness of contraception.[12]

Everyone who takes care of patients knows that there is copious misinformation about contraception and STDs; it may be even more prevalent among adolescents. Frank discussion with health care providers may dispel myths that OCPs cause weight gain, infertility, cancer, strokes, miscarriages, and birth defects. Many adolescents know that OCPs help with dysmenorrhea and abnormal bleeding, but how many know about the other noncontraceptive benefits of OCPs, such as decreasing the rate of ovarian and endometrial cancer or increasing bone density?[13] Dispelling the myths, reinforcing the safety and efficacy, and espousing the noncontraceptive benefits of OCPs may have a positive impact on patient satisfaction and compliance.

Some adolescents may know the specific type of contraception that they want to use before they interact with a health care provider; others may benefit from reviewing a contraceptive menu with a clinician to make the most appropriate choice. For example, patients with gynecologic problems such as chronic anovulation or amenorrhea certainly would benefit from choosing OCPs over long-acting progestins. Patients using hormonal contraception also need to be instructed about the importance of using condoms in conjunction with OCPs to protect from STDs.

The absolute contraindications to OCP use include problems rarely faced by adolescents, such as thrombophlebitis, thromboembolic disorders, cerebrovascular disease, coronary occlusion, markedly impaired liver function, breast cancer, undiagnosed abnormal vaginal bleeding, known or suspected pregnancy, and smoking past the age of 35.[13] The most common concerns for adolescents are pregnancy and hepatitis. These concerns need to be addressed by ruling out pregnancy with a urine or serum pregnancy test and obtaining liver function tests in patients with a history of hepatitis. More adolescents may have relative contraindications to OCP use, including migraine headaches, hypertension, epilepsy, sickle cell disease or sickle C disease, and diabetes mellitus.[13] Patients with absolute and relative contraindications to OCP use need extensive counseling with a physician before initiating therapy to understand potential risks and to evaluate alternative methods of contraception that may be more suited to their needs.

Adequate knowledge about contraceptives is essential for the proper and consistent use of OCPs. Package inserts for OCPs are currently written at the tenth to twelfth grade level.[16] How many adolescents are able to understand the instructions for properly starting and taking OCPs? Will they be able to understand what to do if they miss a pill at different points in the cycle pack? One hopes that most clinicians provide patients with verbal instructions and live demonstrations of the proper use of the pill dispenser before initiating OCP use to increase the likelihood of correct and consistent pill use.

Counseling patients before initiating therapy about potential side effects of OCPs, such as nausea, breast tenderness, and breakthrough bleeding, may improve compliance. Often patients need ongoing dialog with a clinician for reassurance and help with managing the common side effects of OCPs, which usually resolve after the first few cycles of use.[13] Other more serious side effects of OCPs, which require clinical evaluation by the appropriate health care provider, include headaches and hypertension. Both may require discontinuation of OCPs and selection of an alternative form of contraception. Such potential problems will be difficult to monitor if OCPs are available to adolescents over the counter.

PREVENTIVE HEALTH CARE MEASURES

In addition to education and counseling about sexuality and contraception, adolescents receive additional preventive health care measures when they seek medical care for contraceptive services. A general health assessment is performed, including medical history, social history, sexual history, weight, and blood pressure measurement. The physical examination includes a breast exam, abdominal exam, and complete pelvic exam, with an assessment of the external genitalia, vagina, cervix, uterus, and adnexa. Patients can be screened for risky behaviors such as smoking and alcohol and illicit substance abuse, and appropriate interventions and referrals can be made. Other assessments of mental health status can be performed, and further evaluation and treatment may be prescribed. Frank discussion of sexuality and contraceptive needs with the health care provider also may lead to disclosures about physical or sexual abuse. Hepatitis and tetanus vaccines can be provided if indicated.

Papanicolaou smears have side acceptance in the medical community and general public as effective screening tools for premalignant cervical changes. Sexually active adolescents are at increased risk for cervical dysplasia; the incidence of cervical dysplasia in the adolescent age group appears to be increasing.[8] One adolescent clinic reported a 16% incidence of cervical dysplasia first identified by Papanicolaou smear.[9] As in the adult population, Papanicolaou smears in sexually active adolescents can identify patients with premalignant conditions and lead to treatment with a consequent decrease in the incidence of cervical cancer. It has been suggested that the rate of progression of cervical dysplasia to cervical cancer may be increased in young women.[4] However, estimates show that only 12% of all sexually active adolescents have received a Papanicolaou smear.[10] Many clinicians routinely do an annual Papanicolaou smear in adolescents before renewing their OCP prescription. If OCPs were available over the counter without interaction with a clinician, even fewer than 12% of all sexually active adolescents may undergo Papanicolaou smear screening. Clinicians caring for adolescents need to be aware of their patients' sexual practices and initiate Papanicolaou smear screening if appropriate.

Three million cases of STDs are contracted each year by American adolescents. This figure represents 25% of the 12 million cases of STDs identified in the United States each year.[3] More than one-half of these infections occur in young women who are at increased risk compared with their male partners of suffering long-term sequelae of infection. These sequelae include pelvic inflammatory disease, infertility, ectopic pregnancy, and chronic pelvic pain. Such infections, if present during pregnancy, also may lead to poor obstetric outcomes and neonatal complications.

Although they share the same level of sexual activity, American adolescents are much more likely than their European or Canadian counterparts to contract an STD. Prevention and early diagnosis and treatment are the only ways to protect adolescents from the immediate and long-term dangers of STDs. All adolescents need to be informed about the dangers of STDs and about their prevention. The Centers for Disease Control and Prevention recommends that screening tests for the most common bacterial sexually transmitted pathogens—chlamydia and gonorrhea—be performed annually in sexually active adolescents.[1] Screening for hepatitis B may be appropriate in some adolescents, who can be offered the vaccine as a form of protection. Adolescents should be counseled about possible HIV and syphilis screening if deemed appropriate. Many STDs are asymptomatic in young women. In the absence of symptoms, women may not seek appropriate care if antibiotics and OCPs are available without first interacting with a health care provider.

CONCLUSION

All adolescents need ongoing interaction with clinicians, and sexually active adolescents may have an even greater need because of their increased risk of becoming pregnant and acquiring an STD. There are numerous reasons why American adolescents become pregnant and contract STDs at such a high rate, but we must not allow limited access to health care providers to be one of them. Although making OCPs available to adolescents over the counter in theory may increase accessibility, it is not clear that adolescents are able to understand contraindications to their use, appropriate dosing and initiation of therapy, and management of potential side effects and complications. After removal of the currently mandatory interaction with a health care provider to obtain OCPs, many adolescents would fail to benefit from recommended preventive health care strategies. Of importance, they may not be appropriately screened for STDs, including cervical dysplasia. We need to inform adolescents that interaction with physicians and other clinicians may lead to confidential, comprehensive medical care, including gynecologic and contraceptive services.

References

1. Centers for Disease Control and Prevention: Recommendations for the prevention and management of *Chlamydia trachomatis* infections. MMWR 42:RR-12, 1993.
2. Centers for Disease Control: Premarital sexual experiences among adolescent women—United States. MMWR 39:929, 1991.
3. Committee on Prevention and Control of Sexually Transmitted Diseases, Institute of Medicine; Eng TR, Butler WT (eds): The Hidden Epidemic: Confronting Sexually Transmitted Diseases. Washington, DC, National Academy Press, 1996.
4. Crowther ME: Is the nature of cervical carcinoma changing in young women? Obstet Gynecol Surv 50:71, 1994.
5. Delaying pelvic exams to encouarge contraceptive use. Fam Plann Perspect 24:136, 1992.
6. Division of STD/HIV Prevention, Centers for Disease Control and Prevention: Annual Report, 1994. Atlanta, U.S. Department of Health and Human Services, Public Health Service, 1995.
7. Encouraging contraceptive compliance among adolescents. Contracept Rep 1:3, 1992.
8. Hillard PJA, Biro FM, Wildey LS, et al: Cervical dysplasia and human papillomavirus: Evaluation in an adolescent dysplasia clinic. Adolesc Pediatr Gynecol 12:32, 1989.
9. Hillard PJA, Biro FM, Wildey LS, et al: The value of an adolescent dysplasia clinic. Adolesc Pediatr Gynecol 12:32, 1989.
10. Ingra V, Millstein SG: Current status and approaches to improving preventive services for adolescents. JAMA 11:1408–1412, 1993.
11. Malus M, LaChance PA, Lamy L, et al: Priorities in adolescent health care: The teenager's viewpoint. J Fam Pract 25:159, 1987.
12. Mauldon J, Luker D: The effects of contraceptive education on method used at first intercourse. Fam Plann Perspect 28:19, 1996.
13. Speroff L, Darney P: A Clinical Guide to Contraception. Baltimore, Williams & Wilkins, 1992.
14. Orr MT: Private physicians and the provision of contraceptives to adolescents. Fam Plann Perspect 16:83, 1984.
15. van Lunsen RHW, Arnolds HT, van Maris MGM: Choices and changes in contraceptive behaviour: The role of information sources. Patient Educ Counsel 23:197, 1994.
16. Williams-Deane M, Potter LD: Current oral contraceptive use instructions: An analysis of patient package inserts. Fam Plann Perspect 24:111, 1992.
17. Zabin LS, Danter JF, Zelnik M: The risk of adolescent pregnancy in the first months of intercourse. Fam Plann Perspect 11:108, 1979.

Condom Availability in High Schools

J. DENNIS FORTENBERRY, M.D., M.S.

Section of Adolescent Medicine
Department of Pediatrics
Indiana University
Indianapolis, Indiana

Reprint requests to:
J. Dennis Fortenberry, M.D., M.S.
Riley Hospital for Children
702 Barnhill Drive, Room 1740N
Indianapolis, IN 46402

The epidemics of sexually transmitted infections (STI), especially human immunodeficiency virus (HIV), among adolescents have initiated broad public health measures to help adolescents delay initiation of coital sexual activity, to provide education about STI/HIV prevention, and to provide appropriate means to prevent STI/HIV and unintended pregnancy. School-based condom availability programs have been recommended by the American Academy of Pediatrics and the Institute of Medicine as one means to accomplish a specific goal: reduce barriers to obtaining condoms by increasing access to condoms, thereby increasing levels of use.[1,10] Many programs attempt to enhance their potential effectiveness by providing additional counseling for other aspects of risk-reduction, abstinence, and correct condom usage. Despite active opposition, surveys show high levels of support among students and parents for school-based availability programs.[6,13]

Condom availability programs have elicited a number of criticisms. Opponents believe that such programs normalize coital activity and make it appear acceptable behavior for adolescents, thereby diminishing the influence of abstinence or efforts to delay sexual activity.[8,11] High rates of condom failure due to inherent physical limitations of the latex barrier, breakage, slippage, and incorrect use are also cited as justification for opposition of condom availability programs. Some contend that the skills required for successful condom use—communication, assertiveness and refusal—are the same as those required for abstinence-only programs.[8] From this perspective, the latter is a much more appropriate use of resources to encourage a more reliable form of STI/HIV prevention.

Two key issues that are central to the debate are considered in this chapter. First, how successful might school-based condom availability programs be in reducing STI/HIV rates among adolescents? If such programs are ineffective, debate concerning their implementation is a waste of time. Second, do school-based condom availability programs conflict with efforts to promote less risky sexual choices such as abstinence? The unresolved question is whether the two approaches may be complementary rather than contradictory. In an editorial about the lack of developmental focus in adolescent sexuality research, Ehrhardt correctly notes that the debate around these issues has been stagnated for decades and has not advanced despite the scientific evidence.[5] Nevertheless, clinicians must insist on evaluations made by careful appraisal of existing data and demand additional data when the information is inadequate. Both professionally and societally, clinicians are obliged to ask the pertinent questions, confront the truth in the data, and act accordingly, regardless of whether the facts agree with our hopes and ideals.

SCHOOL-BASED CONDOM AVAILABILITY PROGRAMS: EFFECTIVENESS

The first point about condom availability programs that must be clarified is that their effectiveness in reducing STI/HIV infection rates is not established. Data are simply insufficient to allow assessment of whether such programs reduce STI/HIV rates among the target population by increasing consistency of condom use or whether such programs, paradoxically, increase STI/HIV rates by increasing levels of sexual activity.[22] The absence of data allows the debate over condom availability programs to continue without a basis for resolution. Review of the issues related to potential effectiveness, therefore, provides the rationale for such difficult and expensive evaluations.

The theoretical underpinnings of condom availability programs as a public health intervention have been given little attention. The simplest perspective is that condom availability programs overcome age-related inequities in condom access that may occur because commercial or health outlets are difficult to find or because condom acquisition by adolescents is subtly discouraged.[22] School-based programs might reduce such barriers, perhaps making adolescents more amenable to condom use when planning for intercourse. The ability to obtain condoms in settings where trusted persons are available for counseling also has been cited as a reason adolescents feel more comfortable obtaining condoms in school settings.[19]

Whether school-based programs overcome these access barriers is unclear since few programs offer unrestricted, anonymous condom access. In most programs, condoms are distributed by school staff, counselors, or health personnel, often with some form of mandatory counseling and usually with restrictions on the number of condoms provided.[19] Embarrassment or fear of ridicule remain important barriers to condom acquisition in many school-based settings. This may be especially true for adolescent women.[12,14]

This simplistic view of condom availability is too limited to be of use to evaluate the effectiveness of a school-based program. Possession of a condom does not guarantee that the adolescent will use it.

A more useful perspective recognizes the importance of knowledge, values, attitudes, and social norms, especially those reflected by peers. These factors may not be related directly to performance of a specific behavior such as condom use; rather, their influence is mediated through perceived self-efficacy, which integrates knowledge, expectancies about outcomes, past experiences, emotional states, and social influences.[2] Condom use is thus a function of expectations about the outcome of the behavior and expectations about one's ability to perform the behavior. School-based condom availability programs could modify several of the factors related to self-efficacy for condom use. Comprehensive programs such as those advocated by the American Academy of Pediatrics[1] might be expected to provide more effective STI/HIV prevention than programs based on simple condom accessibility. This is an important point since some critics of programs assume that condoms are being distributed to students without regard to whether the student is interested and without providing appropriate information about limitations and correct usage.

In fact, most school programs include condom availability as one part of a larger package of counseling and health services. The services may include school-based health services, comprehensive sexuality education, counseling, and a variety of STI/HIV education programs. In some programs, condoms are available in coin-operated vending machines or in baskets. In others, condoms must be obtained from principals, teachers, or health personnel.[19]

This variability in program structure complicates the evaluation of school-based programs.[22] Programs that take place in schools with comprehensive sexuality education programs distribute significantly more condoms per student than those without such a curriculum. Condom availability within the scope of larger programs may provide students with the knowledge and skills to assure that a condom is present at a coital encounter, its use is successfully negotiated, and that the condom is used correctly. Programs can successfully improve knowledge, attitudes, and correct use of condoms.[23]

INFLUENCE OF CONDOM AVAILABILITY ON ADOLESCENT ABSTINENCE

Similar to the longstanding and now reasonably disproved concern[9,18] that school sexuality curricula increase adolescent sexual activity, the potential influence of school-based condom availability programs on adolescents' sexual activity is a constant feature of critiques of these programs.

This criticism has several elements. First is the concern that condom availability promotes sexual activity by removing fears of pregnancy or infection that otherwise cause an adolescent to avoid coitus until marriage.[11] It is argued that abstinence—the behavior presumed to be available, safe, and effective for adolescent STI/HIV prevention—would therefore be less appealing and less likely to be chosen. Abstinence-only programs are often favored because they presumably have universal availability, are apparently harm-free, and because they are consistent with certain moral and religious codes. The potentially important developmental benefits of sexual exploration and learning that may be inhibited by abstinence-only programs are typically ignored. For widespread implementation as a public health intervention, however, the long-term side effects of such programs have not been evaluated and cannot be presumed to be absent.[5]

Critics also point out that condoms may have significant failure rates for STI/HIV prevention and contraception.[8] If condom availability programs did promote an increase in adolescent sexual activity due to a false sense of protection, increased STI/HIV rates could result. This outcome would have important public health implications if the organism in question was highly transmissible or if the primary effect of condom availability was an increase in number of sexual partners rather than an increase in coital frequency per se.

No data suggest that increased numbers of partners are a result of school-based condom availability programs. The reliability of condoms for STI/HIV prevention is a complex question with no straightforward answers. In vitro studies demonstrate high levels of barrier efficacy for a variety of sexually transmitted organisms, including HIV.[17] Epidemiologic studies show lower rates of cervical dysplasia and carcinoma among women whose male partners are regular condom users.[20] Clinical studies of discordant couples consistently demonstrate that regular condom use reduces the risk of HIV-infection.[7] However, questions remain about the magnitude of protection provided by condoms, given reasonably high levels of slippage and breakage and inappropriate use. Some studies have reported that incidence rates for chlamydia and gonorrhea were no different for subjects reporting regular condom use than for those reporting irregular condom use.[24] Even partial protection provided by condoms, however, could have important implications for the various STI/HIV epidemics.

The assumption that fear of STI/HIV restrains sexual activity requires comment. No study demonstrates that fear of STI/HIV effectively restrains initiation of coital activity or its continuation after initiation. In fact, anxiety may inhibit condom use without necessarily reducing sexual activity.[3] Studies and clinical experience demonstrate that adolescents have intercourse without protection even when aware of the risks and when they would prefer to use protection.[12]

Successful abstinence-only programs have *not* been based primarily on elevating STI/HIV fear to a sufficient level to restrain sexual activity. Rather, these programs focused on goal setting, refusal skills, and supportiveness.[16] The successes of such programs are impressive and should be exploited to their fullest within the context of STI/HIV prevention. Abstinence-only programs cannot provide a complete prevention strategy, however, because a significant proportion of adolescents will invariably become sexually active. Those who favor abstinence-only programs and condemn condom availability programs thus seem to have confused the successes of abstinence programs with the needs for prevention among adolescents who become sexually active. These critics have not provided a strong case for abstinence-only programs in favor of more balanced efforts that encourage delay of sexual activity and promote condom use and contraception when coitus does occur.[15] Such insistence on absolutism in prevention would leave many adolescents without access to important information and services.[4]

SCHOOL-BASED CONDOM AVAILABILITY PROGRAMS: NEEDS

Although controversy over school-based condom availability programs will not be easy to resolve, there are several research objectives that could be helpful:

1. *The effectiveness of school-based condom availability programs for prevention of sexually transmitted infections must be demonstrated.* The extraordinary sense of emergency surrounding STI/HIV prevention can no longer be used as justification for interventions of unproven effectiveness. While the difficulties of conducting such a trial are readily acknowledged, many examples of successful intervention research prove that such projects can be undertaken and useful data obtained.

2. *Condom availability should be evaluated as part of a larger package intended to build prevention self-efficacy.* Comparable schools or school districts could be randomly assigned to add condom availability to a comprehensive STI/HIV prevention program.

3. *The primary outcome should be incident cases of specified sexually transmitted infections rather than indirect indicators such as the number of condoms distributed.* Recent advances in urine-based STI testing should make specimen collection much easier and acceptable to adolescents. Meaningful—rather than statistically significant—changes in STI rates should be expected.

4. *Secondary outcome measures would be overall condom use, use of school-provided condoms, frequency of sex partner change, and frequency of coitus.* Overall condom use should be evaluated because condom availability programs could stimulate increased condom use even if the condoms were obtained from sources other than the school. Innovative measurement of condom use would be required to minimize known difficulties with existing measures.[24]

5. *Abstinence or delay of onset of coitus also should be evaluated as part of a comprehensive package of STI/HIV prevention services.* These evaluations need to have a longitudinal focus, since many sexually experienced adolescents have relatively long periods of little or no coital activity. These periods of abstinence may reasonably qualify as successful outcomes of STI/HIV prevention programs.

CONCLUSION

This chapter has attempted to summarize two related issues that surround the controversy about school-based condom availability programs. These issues are being worked out to some degree through the courts,[20,22] but judicial solutions will not answer the fundamental questions about the role and effectiveness of condom availability programs in larger prevention efforts. The void in information ultimately leaves us only with the role of well-intentioned advocacy.

The unresolved professional and public discourse around the role of schools in STI/HIV prevention is an example of society's willingness to sacrifice the health and well-being of its youth for the sake of retaining long-held mores. Well into the second decade of the HIV epidemic, with HIV as a leading cause of death among young adults, it is this author's opinion that the fact that key public health decisions must be made without appropriate data is a national embarrassment.

ACKNOWLEDGMENT

Writing of this paper was supported in part by the Maternal-Child Health Bureau, Rockville, Maryland (MCJ-189596).

References

1. American Academy of Pediatrics: Condom availability for youth. Pediatrics 95:281–285, 1995.
2. Bandura A: Perceived self-efficacy in the exercise of control over AIDS infection. In Mays VM, Albee GW, Schneider SF (eds): Primary Prevention of AIDS: Psychological Approaches. Newbury Park, CA, Sage Publications, 1989, pp 128–141.
3. Buzwell S, Rosenthal D: Constructing a sexual self: Adolescents' sexual self-perceptions and sexual risk-taking. J Res Adolesc 6:489–513, 1996.
4. Cates W Jr, Hinman AR: AIDS and absolutism—The demand for perfection in prevention. N Engl J Med 327:492–493, 1992.
5. Ehrhardt AA: Our view of adolescent sexuality—A focus on risk behavior without the developmental context. Am J Public Health 86:1523–1525, 1996.
6. Fanburg JT, Kaplan DW, Naylor KE: Student opinions of condom distribution at a Denver, Colorado, high school. J School Health 65:181–185, 1995.
7. Feldblum PJ, Morrison CS, Roddy RE: The effectiveness of barrier methods of contraception in preventing the spread of HIV. AIDS 9(Suppl A):585–593, 1995.
8. Friedman Z, Trivelli L: Condom availability for youth: A high-risk alternative. Pediatrics 97:285, 1996.
9. Furstenberg FF Jr, Moore KA, Peterson JL: Sex education and sexual experience among adolescents. Am J Public Health 75:1331–1332, 1985.
10. Eng TR, Butler (eds): The Hidden Epidemic: Confronting Sexually Transmitted Diseases. Washington, DC, National Academy Press, 1997.

11. Griffin GC: Condoms and contraceptives in junior high and high school clinics: What do you think? Postgrad Med 93:21–38, 1993.
12. Guttmacher S, Lieberman L, Hoi-Chang W, et al: Gender differences in attitudes and use of condom availability programs among sexually active students in New York City public high schools. J Am Med Wom Assoc 50:99–102, 1995.
13. Guttmacher S, Lieberman L, Ward D, et al: Parents' attitudes and beliefs about HIV/AIDS prevention with condom availability in New York public high schools. J School Health 65:101–106, 1995.
14. Hagedorn S: Student views of the school nurse's role in a secondary school condom availability program. J School Health 63:358–360, 1993.
15. Hein K: "Getting real" about HIV in adolescents. Am J Public Health 83:492–494, 1993.
16. Howard M, McCabe JB: Helping teenagers postpone sexual involvement. Fam Plann Perspect 22:21–26, 1990.
17. Judson FN, Ehret JM, Bodin GF, et al: *In vitro* evaluations of condoms with and without nonoxynol 9 as physical and chemical barriers against *Chlamydia trachomatis*, herpes simplex virus type 2, and human immunodeficiency virus. Sex Transm Dis 16:51–56, 1989.
18. Kirby D, Short L, Collins J, et al: School-based programs to reduce sexual risk behaviors: A review of effectiveness. Public Health Rep 109:339–360, 1994.
19. Kirby DB, Brown NL: Condom availability programs in U.S. schools. Fam Plann Perspect 28:196–202, 1996.
20. Mahler K. Condom availability in the schools: Lessons from the courtroom. Fam Plann Perspect 28:75–77, 1996.
21. Slattery ML, Overall JC Jr, Abbott TM, et al: Sexual activity, contraception, genital infections, and cervical cancer: Support for a sexually transmitted disease hypothesis. Am J Epidemiol 130:248–258, 1989.
22. Stryker J, Samuels SE, Smith MD: Condom availability in schools: The need for improved program evaluations. Am J Public Health 84:1901–1906, 1994.
23. Wolk LI, Rosenbaum R: The benefits of school-based condom availability: Cross-sectional analysis of a comprehensive high school-based program. J Adolesc Health 17:184–188, 1995.
24. Zenilman JM, Weisman CS, Rompalo AM, et al: Condom use to prevent incident STDs: The validity of self-reported condom use. Sex Transm Dis 22:15–21, 1995.

Emergency Contraception

MELANIE A. GOLD, D.O.

Department of Pediatrics
Children's Hospital of Pittsburgh
University of Pittsburgh
School of Medicine
Pittsburgh, Pennsylvania

Reprint requests to:
Melanie A. Gold, D.O.
Assistant Professor of Pediatrics
Children's Hospital of Pittsburgh
University of Pittsburgh
School of Medicine
Pittsburgh, PA 15213

Emergency contraception, also called the morning-after-pill or postcoital contraception, is a way to prevent pregnancy after an episode of unprotected intercourse. There are several methods of emergency contraception, including the use of oral high-dose estrogens, high-dose combination estrogen-progestins, high-dose progestins, danazol, mifepristone, and the postcoital insertion of a copper intrauterine device (IUD). In the United States, the most commonly used method of emergency contraception is the Yuzpe method, named for the Canadian obstetrician-gynecologist who first described using high-dose combination oral contraceptive pills for postcoital contraception.[14,15] Six brands of combination oral contraceptive pills marketed in the United States can be prescribed to conform to the Yuzpe regimen (i.e., they contain norgestrel or levonorgestrel as the progestin): Ovral, Lo-Ovral, Nordette, Levlen and the yellow tablets of Triphasil and Tri-Levlen (Table 1). Although oral high-dose progestins are effective for emergency contraception, in the United States the only pill marketed with levonorgestrel, the recommended progestin, is Ovrette, a low-dose formulation. Using this brand for emergency contraception requires two doses of 20 pills each, which must be taken within 48 hours of unprotected intercourse. Most physicians and patients find the prospect of swallowing 40 pills daunting; consequently, the regimen is infrequently used.

THE USE OF COMBINATION PILLS WITH OTHER PROGESTINS

To date, most research on the safety and efficacy of emergency contraceptive pills has been with regimens containing ethinyl estradiol and either norgestrel or levonorgestrel, predominantly because

TABLE 1. Emergency Contraceptive Pill Regimens

Ovral 2 tablets po within 72 hours of unprotected sex, then 2 tablets in 12 hours	Triphasil or Tri-Levlen (yellow tablets ONLY) 4 tablets po within 72 hours of unprotected sex, then 4 tablets in 12 hours
Lo-Ovral, Nordette, or Levlen 4 tablets po within 72 hours of unprotected sex, then 4 tablets in 12 hours	Ovrette (progestin-only method) 20 tablets within 48 hours of unprotected sex, then 20 tablets within 12 hours

these combination pills were the ones available in the 1970s, when most of the research on safety and efficacy was conducted. Theoretically, combination pills with ethinyl estradiol and second-generation progestins such as norethindrone, norethindrone acetate, or ethynodiol diacetate or the newer, third-generation progestins such as desogestrel or norgestimate could be used. However, there has been no research evaluating the efficacy, side effect profile, and safety of these other progestins in combination with ethinyl estradiol as emergency contraceptives.

INDICATIONS FOR USE OF ECPS

Emergency contraceptive pills (ECPs) are indicated any time there has been unprotected sex; they can be used when no preplanned contraceptive method was used, such as when sexual intercourse was unplanned or forced or when a contraceptive method fails, e.g., a condom breaks or a diaphragm slips. ECPs are also indicated if a woman has forgotten to take more than three oral contraceptive pills in a row or it is more than 14 weeks since her last Depo-Provera shot and she had unprotected intercourse. When emergency contraceptive pills are initiated within 72 hours of unprotected intercourse, they reduce the risk of pregnancy by at least 75%.[11] Contraindications to ECPs are thought to be the same as the contraindications to combination oral contraceptives, including thrombophlebitis, myocardial infarction, stroke, breast or estrogen-dependent malignancy, active liver disease, pregnancy, and undiagnosed vaginal bleeding. Since most of these contraindications occur infrequently among adolescents, most adolescent and young women can use ECPs. The most common side effects of ECPs are estrogen-related and include nausea and vomiting, menstrual disturbances, breast tenderness, abdominal cramping, dizziness, headache, and mood change.

ANTIEMETICS AND EXTRA DOSES OF ECPS

Nausea affects 25–60% of ECP users, and vomiting occurs in 11–29%. Vomiting that occurs within 3 hours of ingesting the pills can interfere with complete absorption of the medication and can thus impair efficacy. Some clinicians advocate routinely dispensing an antiemetic to all patients taking ECPs. Others recommend using medical interviewing to screen for antiemetic need; a history of nausea associated with prior oral contraceptive or emergency contraceptive use, or a history of frequent nausea when taking other oral medications would determine if an antiemetic should be prescribed. Some health care providers never dispense an antiemetic to patients taking ECPs. In a study of adolescent health care providers, 46% of physicians who prescribe emergency contraception said they routinely prescribe an antiemetic.[3] When prescribing or recommending an antiemetic, clinicians should advise patients to take the medicine 30 minutes prior to ingesting the ECPs to maximize the antiemetic effect. Patients can buy an over-the-counter antinauseant such as dimenhydrinate (Dramamine, 50 mg tablets) and should be instructed to take 1–2 tablets every 4–6 hours to prevent nausea. If a patient is

TABLE 2. Antiemetics that Can Be Used to Prevent Nausea from Emergency Contraceptive Pills

Nonprescription medications
Dimenhydrinate (Dramamine) 50-mg tablets: 1 to 2 tablets every 4–6 hours
Cyclizine hydrochloride (Marezine) 50-mg tablets: 1 tablet every 4–6 hours
Prescription medications
Trimethobenzamide hydrochloride (Tigan) 250-mg tablets: 1 tablet every 8 hours
Trimethobenzamide hydrochloride (Tigan) 200-mg suppositories: 1 suppository every 8 hours
Promethazine hydrochloride (Phenergan) 25-mg tablets: 1 tablet every 12 hours
Promethazine hydrochloride (Phenergan) 25-mg suppositories: 1 suppository every 12 hours

unable to purchase an antiemetic without a prescription, Tigan or Phenergan can be used (Table 2). For severe vomiting, Phenergan and Tigan are also available in suppository form. However, the use of these prescription antiemetics must be weighed against the risks of extrapyramidal side effects such as dystonic reactions. Such reactions can be frightening to patients and may be perceived as worse than the nausea from the ECPs.

Instead of or in addition to providing an antiemetic, many providers recommend giving patients an extra dose of ECPs to take if they vomit within 3 hours of taking the initial dose. Providing extra pills can be especially important if the patient lives far from the health care provider or pharmacy or if it is difficult for the patient to arrange to get a second dose of medication expediently late at night or on weekends.

TIMING

The chance of pregnancy occurring after a single episode of unprotected intercourse is 20–30% midcycle[15] and 2–4% anytime in the cycle.[10] About half of adolescent medicine specialists who prescribe ECPs use the timing of the menses to determine whether they will prescribe emergency contraception.[3] However, adolescents frequently have irregular menses[12] and often do not remember the exact date of their last menstrual period. In one study of college students receiving emergency contraception, one out of five students had irregular menses.[9] Menstrual irregularity and inability to recall the timing of the last menses can make predicting ovulation for an adolescent difficult and can place her at higher risk of pregnancy because she is unable to predict her fertile time or accurately determine when her period is late. Thus, it seems reasonable to offer ECPs to adolescents after an episode of unprotected intercourse occurring any time during the cycle rather than limiting ECP use to midcycle exposure.

The recommended 72-hour maximum time from unprotected sexual intercourse to initiating emergency contraception was originally chosen by Yuzpe based on his earlier studies demonstrating a reduced efficacy among patients who used the method beyond the 72-hour limit. The theory behind this time frame is based on reproductive physiology; it takes the ovum approximately three days to travel from the ovary to the uterus. However, it can take an additional 2 days for the fertilized ovum to firmly attach to the endometrial lining. Thus, theoretically the time limit of 72 hours may be excessively restrictive and might be extended to 4 or even 5 days after unprotected intercourse. About 57% of adolescent health experts who prescribe ECPs follow the current practice of prescribing it up to 72 hours after unprotected intercourse, 29% prescribe it only to adolescents who seek treatment within 48 hours, and 11% restrict use to 24 hours from exposure.[3] Clearly, such time limitations represent a barrier to increased ECP use. ECP availability will be maximized by routinely dispensing it up to 72 hours after unprotected intercourse. Further research is needed to investigate whether the 72-hour time limit is necessary or if it can be expanded to increase accessibility of emergency contraception.

CONTRAINDICATIONS

The standard contraindications to using ECPs are derived from those for ongoing use of oral contraceptive pills. But is this appropriate? Different risks are associated with taking preparations of low-dose ethinyl estradiol and progestin daily for several months to years versus taking a single high-dose of ethinyl estradiol and levonorgestrel or norgestrel within 12 hours rarely or infrequently. Thrombophlebitis, prior history of a pulmonary embolism, stroke, or deep vein thrombosis are considered absolute contraindications for ongoing contraception with oral low-dose contraceptive pills. However, it is unknown if a single high dose of the same estrogen-progestin combination is as risky. A study of 11 women given the Yuzpe hormonal regimen at midcycle showed no changes in clotting factors.[13] Thus, some health providers have suggested that a history of thrombophlebitis should not be an absolute contraindication to one-time ECP use, especially since pregnancy carries a significantly higher risk to the patient of recurrent thromboembolism. Others have suggested that previous ectopic pregnancy should be an absolute contraindication to ECPs because a few cases of ectopic pregnancy following the use of ECPs have been reported.[7] However, any sexually active young woman with a prior history of ectopic pregnancy will be at high risk of having another ectopic pregnancy. A prior history of ectopic pregnancy, therefore, should not be an absolute contraindication to ECP use but rather should incite caution in the form of closer follow-up 2 weeks after ECP use to ensure that pregnancy—whether intrauterine or ectopic—has been averted. Thus, if an ectopic pregnancy were to result following ECP use, there would be ample time to diagnose it early and to treat it.

ROLE OF A PELVIC EXAMINATION

Since it is currently considered acceptable to delay pelvic examination for up to 3 months for adolescents wishing to initiate oral contraceptives for ongoing contraception, must it be performed prior to prescribing ECPs? The main concern of some clinicians is that the patient will obtain the medication and not return for the 2- to 3-week follow-up visit. Another concern is that the patient may have a sexually transmitted disease (STD) that might otherwise go undetected. If the concern is that a new STD was acquired during the episode of unprotected intercourse, the visit within 72 hours of exposure may be too soon to detect a new infection. Requiring a pelvic examination at the time a patient requests ECPs can act as a barrier to access. In a survey of 133 adolescents, 27% indicated that needing to have a pelvic examination would deter them from seeking ECPs.[2]

MEDICOLEGAL CONSIDERATIONS

Many health care providers have not routinely counseled patients about ECPs or prescribed ECPs because of fears of medicolegal liability. They argue that oral contraceptive pills were not approved by the Food and Drug Administration for emergency use, and they fear excess liability in prescribing a medication for an off-label use. However, on February 25th, 1997, the FDA published a notice in the *Federal Register* affirming that ECPs are safe and effective, and it published the specific protocol for emergency use.[16] Yet, even before FDA approval, health care providers had no need to shy away from prescribing oral contraceptives for emergency contraception because this prescribing pattern had become the standard of care. Many drugs are currently prescribed for indications for which they have never been approved by the FDA. For example, oral contraceptives are commonly prescribed for relief of dysmenorrhea, treatment of hyperandrogenism, and prevention of ovarian cyst formation. Despite the FDA's recent approval, it may be some time before oral contraceptive pills are relabeled or repackaged for emergency contraceptive use. Presently, depending on the brand, patients must purchase a pack of 21 or 28 pills when they only need 4 or 8. Even if the current manufacturers do not repackage their pills as ECPs, the FDA's call for new drug applications will open the likelihood that other companies will market and distribute emergency contraceptive pills, especially since all six available brands are now off patent and may be remanufactured. The sample labeling attached to the FDA's notice in the *Federal Register* has also laid the groundwork for the requirement for proper labeling.

INFORMED CONSENT

Unlike surgical procedures, patients are not legally required to sign informed consent prior to taking medication, even for an off-label indication, unless it is experimental or nonstandard practice. However, many university health services and agencies that provide family planning services have required patients to sign an informed consent that states that the patient understands that use of oral contraceptive pills for emergency contraception is an off-label use, that the method is not 100% effective, and that they understand the potential side effects and risks. A survey found that 25% of adolescent health care providers who prescribe emergency contraception require written informed consent.[3] Since requiring a patient to sign an informed consent implies that the method is dangerous and requires special legal protection for the provider, this requirement may unintentionally act as a barrier to access. A survey of adolescent women found that two-thirds viewed side effects of ECPs and their potential negative impact on future fertility as major barriers to using ECPs.[2] It is questionable whether a signed consent really protects the physician against litigation. However, given the recent FDA approval, this issue is now moot and consent forms are unnecessary.

EQUATING ECPS WITH ABORTION

By the medical definition, pregnancy begins at the time of implantation of a fertilized ovum. Although the mechanism of action of ECPs is not completely understood, it is believed that they work predominantly by changing the receptivity of the endometrial lining to implantation by a fertilized ovum. However, there is also evidence that ECPs may work by preventing ovulation, altering tubal transport of the ovum, and altering the viscosity of cervical mucus, thereby impairing sperm motility. Thus, using a medical definition, ECPs are not abortifacients because they prevent implantation rather than disrupt an already implanted, fertilized ovum. ECPs have been likened to a form of chemical IUD. However, in some religions, life is believed to begin at the time of conception. For individuals believing that fertilization marks the start of a pregnancy, emergency contraceptive pills may be viewed as a form of abortion because they impede implantation and further development of a fertilized ovum. It is imperative that health care providers understand and clearly communicate to patients the way in which emergency contraceptive pills prevent pregnancy after unprotected intercourse. Avoiding the use of emotionally inflammatory terminology and clarifying the mechanism of action will allow patients to make an informed decision about this therapy. ECPs will not disrupt an implanted, fertilized ovum. It is up to the prescribing physician and potential user to decide when life begins and whether preventing implantation is acceptable. In this author's opinion, physicians who are not comfortable prescribing emergency contraceptive pills still have an ethical obligation to inform patients of this option and to refer the patient to another provider if she wishes to obtain the method.

THE EFFECT OF ECPS ON CONTRACEPTIVE PRACTICES OF ADOLESCENTS

Health care providers and patients have expressed concerns regarding the potential misuses of ECPs and the negative impact they could have on future adolescent contraceptive behavior.[3,4] The first question is whether counseling adolescents about the existence of emergency contraception will promote future poor or lax use of preplanned contraceptive methods. This concern can have significant implications for counseling policies. Should all patients, adolescents, and adults be uniformly counseled about ECPs? Should virginal adolescents, who may be the most likely ones to have unplanned and unprotected intercourse, be counseled routinely about emergency contraception, or will this knowledge cause them to be less careful about planning ahead to use contraception when they become sexually active? The answers to these questions are unknown; no nationwide studies of adolescent ECP use have been conducted in the United States. The national survey of adolescent health care providers found that 41% of those who dispense ECPs counsel adolescents routinely about emergency contraception during visits for family planning. In contrast, only 28% of the same physicians counsel about ECPs during visits for routine health care, and even fewer (16%) routinely counsel virginal adolescents.[3] Will knowing that ECPs exist cause a decline in condom use and foster a rise in STDs? No current studies address these questions. One-quarter of adolescent health providers believe that knowing about ECPs would discourage adolescents' compliance with other contraceptive methods.[3] In focus group discussions held with university students, both male and female students voiced concerns about the impact of knowing about ECPs on responsible sexual behavior.[4] Younger students expressed concern that the method would be excessively used and, in general, students felt that easily accessible ECPs would encourage use of this method over barrier methods of contraception and lead to higher rates of sexually transmitted diseases. Both male and female students felt that men might use the availability of ECPs to pressure women into having unprotected intercourse. However, despite these concerns, all the students in the focus groups supported the proposal that clinicians counsel about ECPs and that they dispense ECPs in advance along with condoms in case unprotected exposures occur.[4] Currently, several studies are underway that will evaluate the impact of providing ECPs prophylactically on patients' contraceptive behavior, but none of the studies specifically targets adolescents.

FREQUENT USE OF ECPS

There are three theoretical risks associated with frequent use of ECPs. First, there may be a higher risk of thromboembolism from cumulative estrogen use. Second, there may be an increased incidence of unintended pregnancy if ECPs are used as a regular contraceptive method, because they are less effective than preplanned methods. Third, there may be an increased incidence of STDs if patients fail to use condoms because they think they can rely on ECPs to prevent pregnancy. Regarding the thromboembolic risks, Yuzpe indicated that ECPs could be used as many as 15 times per cycle.[14] Clearly, such use is not recommended, but there is no literature indicating that the risk of thromboembolism is higher with ECP use than during pregnancy. One study documented no change in clotting factors in women after ECP treatment.[13] However, almost one-third of adolescent health experts stated that they believed there might be health risks associated with repeated use of ECPs, and 40% said they might restrict the number of times they would dispense emergency contraception to an individual patient, reflecting physicians' uncertainty about the safety of repeated use of this treatment.[3] There is no literature to document that patients will abuse the method if it is available, and in countries where ECPs are readily available, such as the Netherlands, adolescents have not been reported to over-use the method or to have a higher incidence of STDs.

TERATOGENICITY

There are no controlled studies evaluating the impact of ECPs on early fetal development. In the efficacy and safety studies in which women used ECPs, most of the women who became pregnant terminated their pregnancies. The few who continued their pregnancies to term reported no consistent pattern of fetal anomalies. The only other studies that can be used to extrapolate the teratogenic risk of ECPs to fetal outcome are studies of women who took low-dose oral contraceptive pills during the first trimester because they did not suspect they were already pregnant. Patients who have taken a cycle or two of oral contraceptives in the first trimester of pregnancy are currently advised that the risk is insignificant to warrant terminating the pregnancy, and few teratogenic changes have been reported.[1,5,6,8] Part of the concerns about teratogenicity may stem from the experience with diethylstilbestrol (DES), which in the 1960s was used for both postcoital contraception and stopping preterm labor in the second trimester of pregnancy. DES was later discovered to cause genitourinary anomalies in the fetuses exposed during the second trimester, but it was never found to cause these anomalies when taken as a postcoital contraceptive.

USE OF A URINE PREGNANCY TEST

Given the apparent lack of teratogenicity of emergency contraception, it has been argued that a pregnancy test should not be mandatory prior to prescribing ECPs. However, in most health care facilities, it is considered a standard of care to use a urine pregnancy test prior to dispensing ECPs. The main benefit of detecting a preexisting pregnancy is that ECPs are unnecessary if the patient is already pregnant. Although taking ECPs during pregnancy may not be teratogenic, a patient would still experience the unpleasant side effects. It is crucial to counsel patients that the ECPs will not disrupt a preexisting pregnancy. One of the most challenging scenarios is one in which a patient has two episodes of unprotected intercourse—one 3–10 days earlier and the other within the past 72 hours. There is a 10- to 14-day period from ovulation until a urine pregnancy test can detect a pregnancy. Although a positive pregnancy test would preclude prescribing ECPs, a negative result would not necessarily rule out implantation of a fertilized ovum from the earlier episode of intercourse. In this situation, many health care providers would not offer ECPs. However, one could argue that because ECPs will not disrupt an undetectable preexisting pregnancy and that ECPs are not teratogenic, the greater benefit is that of preventing a pregnancy from the most recent exposure. Taking ECPs in this scenario could reduce the risk of pregnancy from the most current unprotected exposure by 75%. Should the patient be found to be pregnant at the 2-week follow-up appointment, it would not be necessary to recommend termination of the pregnancy for teratogenicity concerns; however, it might not be possible to know if the ECPs failed or if the previous unprotected intercourse exposure had caused the pregnancy.

AVAILABILITY OF EMERGENCY CONTRACEPTION

There has been ongoing discussion among experts regarding making hormonal contraceptive pills available over the counter. Equally, if not more, controversial is the concept of making emergency contraceptive pills available without a prescription. Proponents of making ECPs available believe this will improve access and thus reduce the rate of unintended pregnancies. Opponents believe that over-the-counter status will lead to misuse and abuse. Some believe preferential use of ECPs will result in less use of barrier methods and subsequent higher rates of STDs. Others believe that over-the-counter availability will result in higher adolescent pregnancy rates as a result of improper use or reliance on ECPs as a routine method of contraception. Still others are concerned that ECPs will not be covered by insurance and medical assistance programs. Even in countries where ECPs are easily available, they cannot be purchased without a prescription; thus, the impact of over-the-counter status of ECPs on adolescents' contraceptive behavior remains unknown.

SUMMARY

Data indicate that emergency contraceptive pills are safe and effective for adolescents and are underutilized in the United States. The FDA has recognized this by approving certain oral contraceptive pills for use as ECPs. As ECPs become more widely used, their impact on pregnancy and STD rates and other contraceptive behaviors will be clarified.

References

1. Braken MB: oral contraceptives and congenital malformations in offspring: A review and meta-analysis of the prospective studies. Obstet Gynecol 76:552–557, 1990.
2. Gold MA, Miller R: Adolescent and young women's attitudes towards, knowledge about, and perceived barriers to using emergency contraception [abstract]. J Adolesc Health 29:144, 1997.
3. Gold MA, Schein A, Coupey SM: Emergency contraception: A national survey of adolescent health experts. Fam Plann Perspect 29:15–19,24, 1997.
4. Harper C, Ellerston C: Knowledge and perceptions of emergency contraceptive pills among college-age population: A qualitative approach. Fam Plann Perspect 27:149–154, 1995.
5. Janerich DT, Piper JM, Glebatis DM: Oral contraceptives and congenital limb-reduction defects. N Engl J Med 291:697–700, 1974.
6. Kaufman RL: Birth defects and oral contraceptives. Lancet 1:1396, 1973.
7. Kubba AA, Guillebaud J: Case of ectopic pregnancy after postcoital contraception with ethinyloestradiol-levonorgestrol. BMJ 287:1343–1344, 1983.
8. Nora JJ, Nora AH: Can the pill cause birth defects? N Engl J Med 291:731–732, 1974.
9. Schilling LH: An alternative to the use of high dose estrogens for postcoital contraception. J Am Coll Health 27:247–249, 1979.
10. Tieze C: Probability of pregnancy resulting from a single unprotected coitus. Fertil Steril 11:485–488, 1960.
11. Trussell J, Ellerston C, Stewart F: The effectiveness of the Yuzpe regimen of emergency contraception. Fam Plann Perspect 28:58–64,87, 1995.
12. Widholm O, Kantero RL: Menstrual pattern of adolescent girls according to chronologic age and gynecologic age. Acta Obstet Gynecol Scand 14:19–29, 1971.
13. Webb A, Taberner D: Clotting factors after emergency contraception. Adv Contracept 9:75–82, 1993.
14. Yuzpe AA, Lancee WJ: Ethinylestradiol and dl-norgestrel as a postcoital contraceptive. Fertil Steril 9:932–936, 1977.
15. Yuzpe AA, Thurlow HJ, Ramzy I, Leyshon JI: Postcoital contraception—a pilot study. J Reprod Med 13:53–58, 1974.
16. Prescription drug products: Certain combination oral contraceptives for use as postcoital emergency contraception. Federal Register 62:8610–8612, 1997.

Adolescents and HIV: Controversies Old and New

S. KENNETH SCHONBERG, M.D.
NEAL D. HOFFMAN, M.D.

Albert Einstein College of Medicine
Division of Adolescent Medicine
Montefiore Medical Center
Bronx, New York

Reprint requests to:
S. Kenneth Schonberg, M.D.
Division of Adolescent Medicine
Montefiore Medical Center
111 East 210th Street
Bronx, NY 10467

During the past 20 years issues relating to the acquired immune deficiency syndrome (AIDS) epidemic have uniquely captured the attention of the medical community and the general public. Discussions of these issues have been controversial and heated. Many factors have contributed to both the extent of the attention paid to the AIDS epidemic and the vehemence that has characterized much of the debate.

Among the factors that have drawn attention were the fatal nature of this new contagious illness and the initial uncertainties about its etiology and mode of transmission. We were some years into the epidemic before the etiologic agent, human immune deficiency virus (HIV), was determined and the most and least likely modes of transmission clearly defined. Did the afflicted represent a threat to public health? Did we need to find out who they were and exclude them from schools, workplaces, and playing fields? Should infected health care workers and, in particular, surgeons be precluded from practice? Should infected teachers be allowed into the classroom? Should infected children be allowed to attend school or day care or even live in the community?

The first waves of the epidemic most heavily affected adults, specifically injection drug abusers and gay men. Drug abusers had little power to influence the decisions of either the body politic or the medical community, whereas gay men were in the initial stages of exercising their political power and insisting on their civil rights. For gay men this stigmatizing and ultimately devastating epidemic could not have come at a worse time. Neither group had reason to trust that either the medical community or the political leadership would consistently act in their best interest. Consequently, initial debates about issues such as testing and confidentiality were guided as much by public health concerns as they were by issues of civil rights and a legacy of distrust of politicians and physicians. The debate was fueled by subsequent inactivity by government and community agencies, reflecting expressed views that both drug abuse and homosexuality were voluntary immoral acts. Hence, those infected with HIV or at risk of becoming infected were not considered worthy of society's full attention or deepest concern for their civil or privacy rights.

For many years we had no effective treatments for HIV infection. If there were no effective treatments, why should anyone seek testing? Would the knowledge that one had an untreatable, "universally fatal" illness be better than not knowing and be worth the risks of possible disclosure? As the confidentiality of test results could not be assured, why risk disclosure, discrimination, loss of housing and employment, and ostracization?

Much has changed over the two decades. Effective and possibly even curative treatment is now available. Advances in treatment have increased the urgency and importance of identifying infected individuals, and HIV-infected people have more reason to seek diagnosis and care. The epidemic has spread well beyond the groups initially involved and includes many adolescents, both male and female, engaged in heterosexual intercourse. Although it has been years since the last public rally was held to exclude an HIV-infected child from school, discrimination against the infected certainly continues, although it is now less vocal and more subtle. As some controversies have quieted, others have arisen, and it is worthwhile to elaborate the issues surrounding HIV infection and adolescents that remain unresolved:

- Who should be tested?
- What level of counseling is necessary as a prerequisite for testing?
- May adolescents legally consent to testing?
- What are the requisites and limitations of confidentiality, particularly as they relate to the issues of parental and partner notification?
- What constitutes the best treatment options for adolescents?
- How may adolescents participate in research treatment protocols when parental consent is unavailable?

WHOM TO TEST

In the early years of the epidemic, HIV infection among adolescents was uncommon, and testing was recommended only when an ill adolescent presented with a clinical picture suggestive of underlying immunodeficiency. Clinicians tested when they encountered generalized lymphadenopathy, tuberculosis, or opportunistic infections. Later, as HIV infection became more common in this age group, testing was recommended not only for young people with a clinical picture suggestive for AIDS but also for adolescents who were members of "high-risk groups," i.e., injection drug users, prostitutes, male homosexuals, and recipients of blood transfusions before 1985.[1] The designation "high-risk groups" was changed to "high-risk behaviors" to avoid unfair stigmatization of groups of people and to indicate more accurately that particular behaviors placed adolescents in the path of the virus. A history of repetitive episodes of sexually transmitted diseases—in particular, conditions characterized by ulcerative lesions (syphilis and herpes)—was added to the list of indications to recommend testing.[24] Reports of an association between the use of crack-cocaine and HIV infection, almost certainly secondary to the sexual practices necessary to support a drug habit—added another indication for testing.[9] Recent data suggest that assessment for possible HIV infection should be far more common than it has been.

Although adolescents account for less than 1% of total reported cases of AIDS, over 20% of cases occur in young adults between ages 20 and 29.[5] Many young adults diagnosed with AIDS contracted HIV infection during adolescence. There are no data from national cross-sectional studies about the prevalence of HIV infection among adolescents. However, studies of selected populations of young people give some indication of the extent of infection among the adolescent population. Among applicants to the Job Corps screened between 1987 and 1990, the prevalence of HIV infection was 3.6/1000.[6] Among 20-year-old patients receiving care at a sexually transmitted disease clinic in Baltimore between 1987 and 1989, 21/1000 were found to be HIV-positive.[18] Among adolescents aged 18 to 19 years receiving care at a hospital in Washington, D.C., the rate of HIV infection was 5.6/1000.[8] In a small study of homeless and runaway youth, 16% of those aged 18–21 years were HIV-positive.[25] Among adolescents who have been diagnosed with AIDS to date, the male:female ratio approximates 1.7:1 compared with an adult ratio of 6:1. It is currently estimated that 25% of people newly infected with HIV are aged 22 years or younger.[20]

A combination of factors indicates that it is no longer sufficient to recommend testing for HIV only to adolescents who have suggestive symptoms and who give a history of having engaged in what have been traditionally characterized as high-risk behaviors. First, available data demonstrate that HIV infection among adolescents is no longer a rarity. Next, among the high proportion of female adolescents who have been found to be infected, the behavior that put them in the path of the virus was heterosexual activity with a partner whom they often did not know to be either infected or at special risk of infection. Finally, HIV transmission has become a treatable illness, and treatment will continue to improve, placing a premium on the early identification of infected people.

In our opinion, providers should include both homosexual and heterosexual experiences in their risk assessment, and testing should be offered to all sexually active adolescents, a description that applies to roughly one-half of the population. The virus is sufficiently prevalent within the adolescent and young adult populations, and there is no reliable way for a person to know that a sex partner is not infected. Accepting the need to broaden the indications for testing adolescents will affect both current, less aggressive practices and the extent to which comprehensive pretest counseling has been a standard of care.

HOW MUCH PRETEST COUNSELING IS REQUIRED?

Standard practice has been that adolescents require extensive counseling before being offered HIV testing and additional counseling after a positive or negative result has been determined. In particular, the emphasis on pretest counseling stands in sharp contrast to the vast majority of other screening tests performed for adolescents, such as urinalysis, blood counts, tuberculin tests, and tests for sexually transmitted diseases. Consent for testing is often assumed, and there is little conversation about the implications of a positive finding unless and until some pathology is discovered.

Beyond an assessment of risk for HIV, recommendations for the components of pretest counseling have included discussion of sexual orientation and practices; provision of education about HIV and routes of transmission; emphasis on reduction of subsequent risk with skills training; assessment for the availability of a supportive adult if the test is positive; determination of risk for severe depression and suicidality if results are positive; explanation of confidentiality and its limits, including the potential for disclosure and resultant discrimination; and, of great importance, determination that consent for testing was truly voluntary and informed.[22] Although there is no argument that adolescents benefit from a discussion of these topics, such comprehensive counseling places a heavy time burden on the practitioner. Beyond the burden of time is the implication that such counseling requires special knowledge and special skills. Thus it is best left to trained HIV counselors and should not be attempted by house officers or practitioners who lack the necessary expertise. An additional concern is that the emphasis on requisite counseling stands in contrast to the current availability of home collection systems that allow a person to forward a blood sample to a commercial laboratory and receive results by telephone without a health care provider as an intermediary.

Despite the admitted value of counseling, educating, and training adolescents, now may be the time to reconsider the standards for pretest counseling. If we are committed to the early identification of infected adolescents and if we believe that testing should be offered to all adolescents who have unprotected intercourse, we must promote testing practices that are compatible with the skills of the majority of practitioners and that do not require excessive time. The message must be that large numbers of adolescents require assessment for HIV and that such assessment is within the capabilities of all physicians. We must reconsider which components of pretest counseling remain essential and which serve as an obstacle to receiving necessary assessment rather than as a benefit or protection. We must simultaneously provide the resources and training for providers that will allow them to accomplish the testing process. The facilitation of testing must be accomplished without an assault on the principle of informed consent, which in some ways assumes unique importance in treating adolescents with HIV infection.

MAY ADOLESCENTS LEGALLY CONSENT TO TESTING?

Older adolescents—i.e., those who have reached their 18th birthday—are considered adults for the purpose of receiving medical care and may consent to all evaluations and treatments. Adolescents below the age of 18 are minors, and their ability to consent to care is defined by specific statutes in the jurisdiction in which they seek care. Although all states allow minors to receive evaluation and treatment for sexually transmitted diseases without parental knowledge or consent, not all states have defined HIV as a sexually transmitted disease for the purposes of consent to care. However, at this time most states have regulations that specifically allow minors to consent to HIV testing and treatment. In the absence of regulations that either permit or forbid the testing of minors on their own consent, the health care provider must make a judgment as to what course serves the adolescent's best interest. Affecting that judgment are factors such as the adolescent's maturity, his or her relationship with family, the likelihood that the adolescent will be able to deal with the consequences of a positive test without family support, and the potential that seeking parental consent will reveal or imply to the family sexual or drug use behaviors and thus result in harm to the adolescent. In most circumstances the potential benefits of testing far outweigh whatever may be gained from insisting on parental involvement and consent. Without laws to the contrary or compelling reasons to involve the family, it is usually best to proceed on the basis of the adolescent's consent alone, while continuing to encourage the adolescent to involve another adult whom they trust for support through the testing process.

WHAT ARE THE LIMITS OF CONFIDENTIALITY?

The revelation that a person is infected with HIV continues to be associated with discrimination in employment, education, housing, athletics, and social relationships.

There is little question, therefore, that confidentiality should be vigorously protected. However, there are two circumstances in which the limits and advisability of confidentiality are uncertain in caring for an HIV-positive adolescent. Should the fact that an adolescent is infected with HIV be shared with the parents? Should it be shared with identifiable sexual partners?

Certainly it is best for any adolescent faced with the problems of coping with a chronic and potentially fatal illness to have the assistance of supportive parents. The psychologic stress of being ill, the logistics of receiving care, the need for assistance in making treatment decisions, and the requirements of planning for an uncertain future are made less difficult for adolescents as well as adults by the support of significant others. Unfortunately, some adolescents who contract HIV infection have been alienated from their parents, whereas others, who have reasonable relationships with their families, are unable, unwilling, or afraid to reveal their HIV status or the behaviors that placed them at risk to their parents. Consequently, they may request or demand that their parents not be informed and resist all attempts at reconciliation with their families and all offers of assistance with voluntarily revealing their HIV status.

As with issues of consent, statutes in particular jurisdictions may mandate one course of action or another. Laws in some states prohibit any disclosure of the adolescent's HIV status without the consent of the adolescent, whereas in other states disclosure to parents is required on request, when the adolescent is unemancipated, or when the patient is below the age of 16. Without specific direction from the law, clinical personnel must decide whether it is better to honor the adolescent's wishes or to notify parents despite the adolescent's objections. Honoring the adolescent's wishes runs the risk of leaving him or her without mature support in making difficult decisions and facing emotional stress. Ignoring the adolescent's wishes risks creating an adversarial relationship and possibly alienating the adolescent. At times adolescents who are unable to involve their families find support from other relatives or trusted adults. Without such supports it is often tempting for clinical personnel to attempt to fill the vacuum and risk obliterating the necessary boundaries between health care provider and patient.

No single course of action can be recommended for all adolescents in all circumstances. The health care provider must make an individualized decision based on the maturity and particular circumstances of the patient and what is known about the parents and significant others. In reaching this decision, the provider must take seriously the adolescent's perception of parental response to revelation. Anxieties about disclosures to parents are often quite accurate. Many families respond intensely and unfavorably to the news that their child is HIV-positive, homosexual, or abusing drugs. The result of such disclosures may well be further alienation or abandonment rather than increased support.

An equally controversial and difficult decision concerns the disclosure that an adolescent is infected with HIV to a sexual partner. In general, the purposes of disclosure are twofold: to assist the sexual partner in reducing ongoing risk of HIV infection through safer sexual behavior or abstinence and to encourage the person to be tested for HIV infection to access necessary health care. Clearly every effort should be made to enable the patient to notify all sexual partners voluntarily. The health care provider may be bound by local statutes that either mandate or forbid such notification. The dilemma arises when the patient adamantly and persistently refuses to inform sexual partners and the law is nondirective. Involuntary disclosure will certainly alienate the patient and may place the patient at risk of serious physical harm. Such disclosure may be in direct violation of the informed consent that allowed the HIV testing. In obtaining informed consent, the health care provider often promises that all results will be strictly confidential. An additional concern in many clinical situations is that a program's practice of involuntary disclosure will become well known to the population that the program hopes to engage in care and may discourage other young people from seeking care at that site. Finally, the only way of finding out about the sexual practices of patients and the identity of their partners is through their honest responses to queries. That honesty is jeopardized when we use the information to notify sexual partners against the wishes of the adolescent patient. The arguments against involuntary disclosure are quite compelling.

And yet there is something unsettling about knowing that an uninformed sexual partner continues to be exposed to a potentially fatal disease. The following factors make it most difficult to honor promises of confidentiality and to place programmatic concerns ahead of concerns for the welfare of an unsuspecting at-risk third party:

- HIV-positive patients often return for care, having contracted other sexually transmitted diseases that signify continued unprotected intercourse. It is the rare adolescent who consistently uses condoms.
- Many young women who are infected with HIV were unaware that their partner was infected.
- HIV infection can be prevented, and it is now a potentially treatable illness, particularly when diagnosed in the early stages; seeking early diagnosis, however, depends on awareness of risk.

Certainly health care providers should actively and aggressively seek the patient's permission to notify sexual partners and offer assistance and options for how to do so. In our experience, the overwhelming majority of youth, with sufficient education and support, are able to make the disclosure or will give permission for disclosure. However, after failure to obtain the patient's permission within a reasonable time, there is an obligation to inform unsuspecting sexual partners and to provide them with HIV risk reduction counseling and HIV testing. Barring a clear threat of physical violence, the option presented to the patient is no longer whether to inform a sexual partner but rather how and when. We reach this conclusion with neither comfort nor certainty, but in our opinion it represents the best choice in a difficult situation.

TREATMENT CONTROVERSIES

The treatment of HIV infection has improved markedly with the introduction of several new antiretroviral medications, the most potent of which are the protease inhibitors. Combining nucleoside-analog reverse transcriptase inhibitors (zidovudine is the prototype) with any of the currently available protease inhibitors or with a third class of medications known as nonnucleoside reverse transcriptase inhibitors has provided clinicians with a more diverse armamentarium to curb the progression of disease.[2] The reported success to date in suppressing viral replication, relieving symptoms, and prolonging survival substantiates the claim that HIV infection is now a chronic illness.

However, the introduction of new treatments has been accompanied by controversies, not the least of which is the expense of the medications, which are not readily reimbursed through all insurance systems and not available to the developing world where 90% of HIV-infected persons live. Although the newest medications are approved for use by adolescents, they have not been formally studied in this age group because of limited adolescent participation in the clinical trial system. It is reasonable to presume that most adolescents will respond in the same manner as adults because most were infected during their teen years when their immune systems were fully mature. However, approximately 15% of adolescents with HIV have congenital infection and may have a unique disease course that is comparable neither to that of adults nor to that of younger children.[10,19] Little is known about choosing and dosing antiretroviral medications for this growing subpopulation of long-term survivors.

A current uncertainty is when to begin treatment. None of the large clinical trials has included patients with CD4-cell counts above 500/mm^3—that is, patients early in the course of HIV infection. Based on research demonstrating that viral replication and CD4-cell destruction are active processes early in the course of the infection, most researchers recommend early intervention.[11] This strategy has been further substantiated by the retrospective finding within a large cohort of HIV-infected persons that the number of viral copies in the blood, commonly known as the viral load, is directly correlated with the likelihood of disease progression.[16]

With the advent of viral load testing, clinicians are now able to gauge more accurately the efficacy of a particular antiretroviral regimen, because changes in viral load occur sooner than changes in CD4-cell count or clinical status.[23] It remains to be determined exactly how long viral replication must be suppressed with antiretroviral medication. Current opinion suggests that the earliest a patient should consider tapering or discontinuing daily medication is after 2 years of treatment.[17] The recommendation of a minimal 2-year course of treatment presents a significant challenge to any patient, but certainly to an adolescent infected with HIV, who may lack developmentally a sense of future orientation or cognitive understanding of how the medications work or face social issues of disclosure or transient living situations. Like adolescents with cancer who face long years of chemotherapy to effect a cure, adolescents with HIV need strong familial and social supports to ensure successful treatment.

Significant advances have been made in the prevention of AIDS-related complications, such as *Pneumocystis carinii* pneumonia (PCP) and disseminated *Mycobacterium avium* complex infection (DMAC), which are responsible for much of the wasting seen in patients with AIDS, and blindness due to cytomegalovirus (CMV) disease. The results are improved quality of life and prolonged survival for many patients with advanced disease. These advances have contributed significantly to the recently documented decline in HIV-related deaths.[5] Current recommendations about prophylaxis rely on the monitoring of CD4-cell count, although the role of viral load testing as an indicator is under investigation.[13] It remains unclear whether one can discontinue chemoprophylaxis for opportunistic infections when antiretroviral treatment results in a significant increase in CD4-cell count. Reports of PCP at CD4-cell counts greater than 200/mm^3, the usual threshold for predicting susceptibility, have resulted in recommendations that it may be prudent to continue prophylactic regimens until the CD4 count is higher.

Since 1994, the role of zidovudine has assumed new importance in reducing the risk that a pregnant woman will transmit HIV to her infant. Well-controlled studies have shown that zidovudine, started in the second trimester and given through delivery and then to the infant for 6 weeks, reduces the HIV transmission rate by two-thirds (from 25% to 8%).[7] Further information will soon be available through case-controlled studies of the safety and efficacy of other medication regimens during pregnancy, with new recommendations beyond zidovudine soon to follow.[3] The choice of an antiretroviral regimen, including zidovudine alone, to prevent perinatal transmission is not without controversy. It potentially jeopardizes the well-being of the pregnant woman for the benefit of the fetus, because monotherapy for HIV infection is no longer the standard of care. The goal remains to choose a regimen that will minimize adverse effects on the mother and maximize the health of both mother and fetus. This issue is particularly germane to adolescent women with HIV infection, who often need to make decisions about pregnancy. Of note, one-fourth of the women studied in the zidovudine trial were younger than 22 years.

The most controversial issue concerning treatment has resulted from an improved understanding of the sexual transmission of HIV infection.[21] The risk of becoming infected with HIV after unprotected vaginal or anal intercourse is estimated to be 1 in 300, equivalent to the risk of becoming infected after occupational exposure through a needlestick injury. With the documented efficacy of early antiretroviral therapy after occupational exposure and of antiretroviral therapy during the acute phase of HIV infection, also known as primary infection, researchers have begun to speculate about the role of antiretroviral therapy following sexual exposure to HIV infection.[4,14,15] The idea of a "morning after" antiretroviral cocktail is fraught with anxieties about undoing a decade and a half of prevention strategies—if, in fact, it results in an increase in unprotected sexual behavior. This argument is similar to the one advanced about emergency or postcoital contraception. Moreover, the practice of intermittent dosing of antiretroviral therapy may create an even more diverse pool of viruses and increase the difficulty of treating persons who become infected with potentially resistant viral strains.[12,27] The group for whom this controversial postcoital treatment is most germane is adolescents, for whom sexual transmission is the predominant exposure route for HIV infection.[26]

Yet another controversy related to the treatment of HIV infection in adolescents is that new and promising therapeutic regimens are initially available only through participation in research protocols. Because minors are precluded from participation in any but minimal-risk research without parental consent, the younger adolescent who has chosen not to reveal his or her diagnosis to the family will not be allowed to receive newer treatments. Currently, proposals are being advanced to allow participation of minors in therapeutic trials without parental consent while protecting them against unscrupulous experimentation. Components of such proposals include assessment of the adolescent's ability to understand available options and the consequences of accepting or refusing specific therapy; the provision of guidance from an adult not directly involved in the research; and community approval of research involving minors. The resolution of this issue awaits official sanction of some method of substituting for parental consent.

CONCLUSION

Because of the unique status of adolescents as neither children nor adults, their health care has always been characterized by therapeutic, legal, and ethical uncertainties. These uncertainties have been compounded by the controversies surrounding the care of patients of all ages who are infected with HIV. Two decades of debate have resolved some of the controversies, but new ones arise as a result of therapeutic advances and changes in our perspectives and understanding of the illness. We have attempted to delineate the more important of the current controversies, with occasional thoughts about the best answers to difficult questions. We hope that the controversies herein will achieve timely resolution. Dealing with the controversial is intellectually stimulating—part of the allure and excitement of medicine. Certainly resolution of controversy is better for patients.

References

1. American Academy of Pediatrics, Task Force on Pediatric AIDS: Adolescents and human immunodeficiency virus infection: The role of the pediatrician in prevention and intervention. Pediatrics 92:626, 1993.
2. Carpenter CC, Fischl MA, Hammer SM, et al: Antiretroviral therapy for HIV infection in 1996: Recommendations of an international panel. JAMA 276:146, 1996.
3. Centers for Disease Control and Prevention: Recommendations of the US Public Health Service Task Force on the use of zidovudine to reduce perinatal transmission of human immunodeficiency virus. MMWR 43:1, 1994.
4. Centers for Disease Control and Prevention: Provisional public health service recommendations for chemoprophylaxis after occupational exposure to HIV. MMWR 45:468, 1996.
5. Centers for Disease Control and Prevention: Trends in AIDS incidence, deaths and prevalence—United States 1996. MMWR 46:165, 1997.
6. Coates TJ, Faigle M, Stall RD: Does HIV prevention work for men who have sex with men? Report from the Office of Technology Assessment. San Francisco, University of California, Center for AIDS Prevention Studies, 1995.
7. Connor EM, Sperling RS, Gelber R, et al: Reduction of maternal-infant transmission of human immunodeficiency virus type I with zidovudine. N Engl J Med 331:1173, 1994.
8. D'Angelo LJ, Geston PR, Luban NLC, Gayle HD: Human immunodeficiency virus infection in urban adolescents: Can we predict who is at risk? Pediatrics 88:982, 1991.
9. Fullilove MT, Fullilove RE: Intersecting epidemics: Black teen crack use and sexually transmitted disease. J Am Med Wom Assoc 44:146, 1989.
10. Grubman S, Gross E, Lerner-Weiss N, et al: Older children and adolescents living with perinatally acquired human immunodeficiency virus infection. Pediatrics 95:657, 1995.
11. Ho DD, Neuman AU, Perelson AS, et al: Rapid turnover of plasma virion and CD lymphocytes in HIV-1 infection. Nature 373:123, 1995.
12. Hu DJ, Dondero TJ, Rayfield MA, et al: The emerging genetic diversity of HIV. JAMA 275:210, 1996.
13. Kaplan JE, Masur H, Holmes KK, et al: UPHS/ISDA Guidelines for the prevention of opportunistic infections in persons infected with human immunodeficiency virus: Introduction, overview, and disease-specific recommendations. Clin Infect Dis 21(Suppl 1):S1, 1995.
14. Katz MH, Gerberding JL: Postexposure treatment of people exposed to the human immunodeficiency virus through sexual contact or injection-drug use. N Engl J Med 336:1097, 1997.
15. Kinloch-de Loes S, Hirschel BJ, Hoen B, et al: A controlled trial of zidovudine in primary human immunodeficiency virus infection. N Engl J Med 333:408, 1995.
16. Mellors JW, Kingsley LA, Rinaldo CR, et al: Quantification of HIV-1 RNA in plasma predicts outcome after seroconversion. Ann Intern Med 122:573, 1995.
17. Perelson AS, Neumann AU, Markowitz M, et al: HIV-1 dynamics in vivo: Virion clearance rate, infected cell-life span, and viral generation time. Science 271:582, 1996.
18. Quin TC: Evaluation of HIV epidemic among patients attending STD clinics. J Infect Dis 165:541, 1992.
19. Rodgers AS, Futterman D, Levin L, D'Angelo L: A profile of human immunodeficiency virus-infected adolescents receiving health care services at selected sites in the United States. J Adolesc Health 19:401, 1996.
20. Rosenberg PS, Biggar RJ, Goedert JJ: Declining age of HIV infection in the United States. N Engl J Med 330:789, 1994.
21. Royce RA, Sena A, Cates W, Cohen MS: Sexual transmission of HIV. N Engl J Med 336:1072, 1997
22. Ryan C, Futterman D (eds): Lesbian and Gay Youth: Care and Counseling. Adolesc Med State Art Rev 8:315, 1997.
23. Saag MS, Holodniy M, Kuritzkes DR, et al: HIV viral load markers in clinical practice. Nature Med 2:625, 1996.
24. Stamm WE, Handsfield H, Rompalo SM, et al: The association between genital ulcer disease and the acquisition of HIV infection in homosexual men. JAMA 260:1429, 1988.
25. Stricof RL, Kennedy JT, Natell TO, et al: HIV seroprevalence in a facility for runaway and homeless adolescents. Am J Public Health 81:50, 1988.
26. United States Department of Health and Human Services: HIV/AIDS Surveillance Report, Year-end ed. Vol. 8, 1996.
27. Vella S: Clinical implications of resistance to antiretroviral drugs. AIDS Clin Care 9:45, 1997.

Medical Abortions in Adolescents: Should Pediatricians Perform Them?

MITCHELL D. CREININ, M.D.

Department of Obstetrics, Gynecology and Reproductive Sciences
University of Pittsburgh School of Medicine
Magee-Womens Hospital
Pittsburgh, Pennsylvania

Reprint requests to:
Mitchell D. Creinin, M.D.
University of Pittsburgh School of Medicine
Department of Obstetrics, Gynecology and Reproductive Sciences
Magee-Womens Hospital
300 Halket Street
Pittsburgh, PA 15213-3180

Most evaluations of abortion acceptability include women 18 years of age or older. However, in the United States more than 1 million teenage women become pregnant annually.[19] In other words, about one of every 10 women younger than 20 gets pregnant per year.[19] More than 70,000 abortions were performed in 1991 in women younger than 18.[5] Thus, an understanding of this method of resolving unwanted pregnancy in adolescent women is needed. Unlike most adults, adolescents often have different social pressures, living conditions (with parents), and financial limitations. In reality, though, many adults do not have future planning or coping skills that mature with their chronologic age.

The availability of abortion services to adolescents has become more restricted in the past decade. Multiple states have passed and enacted laws mandating parental consent so as to enforce the importance of the family and support of the parents in making such important decisions. These laws allow a woman younger than 18 to obtain a court order (judicial bypass) stating that she is considered by the court to be mature enough to make such a decision on her own or that she faces grave physical or psychologic harm if she is forced to reveal the pregnancy to her parent(s). Even though such laws may have good intention, they are too little, too late. The involvement of the parents in adolescent sexuality needs to occur before pregnancy and not as a result of pregnancy. Such laws have been shown to be of no benefit and only serve to delay the teen from obtaining her desired abortion.[17] The American Academy of Pediatrics strongly opposes such limitations.[1]

TABLE 1. Drugs Used for Medical Abortion Regimens

	Mifepristone	Methotrexate	Misoprostol
Type of drug	Antiprogestin	Antimetabolite	Prostaglandin analogue
Usual dose	600 mg	50 mg/m^2	400–800 μg
Route of administration	Oral	Intramuscular	Intravaginal or oral

This concept of delay is important when a woman is facing the decision between medical or surgical abortion. A medical abortion in the United States is a safe and effective option only through 49 days from the last menstrual period. Surgical abortion can be performed as early as the pregnancy test is positive[9] and does not have an upper limit of 49 days' gestation. Thus, for any woman to have the option of medical abortion, she must be aware of her pregnancy early in gestation and have access to abortion services without limitations such as parental consent laws.

This chapter does not focus on how or why an adolescent chooses to have an abortion as opposed to continuing the pregnancy. Rather it focuses on the decision that comes next: should the abortion be performed medically or surgically? The following section describes the use of mifepristone, methotrexate, and misoprostol for medical abortion (Table 1).

HOW A MEDICAL ABORTION WORKS

Mifepristone (RU 486)

Progesterone, as suggested by its name ("pro-gestation"), is fundamentally important for sustaining an early pregnancy. If progesterone support is withdrawn, the embryo is expelled by a prostaglandin-mediated mechanism. Inhibition of progesterone effects can be accomplished by preventing its synthesis or blockade of its action at the receptor. Mifepristone (RU 486), a derivative of norethindrone, works at the progesterone receptor as a "dud" hormone. By binding tightly to the receptor without activating it, it prevents the action of progesterone and acts as an "antiprogestin." Unfortunately, because of its use as an abortifacient, mifepristone has been falsely labeled as an abortion pill. As an antiprogestin, it has many other applications, including emergency contraception, a use that ironically prevents the need for abortion.

Inhibition of progesterone in early pregnancy causes the trophoblast to shear off the endometrium. Mifepristone also stimulates prostaglandin production by the myometrium and increases the sensitivity of the uterus to prostaglandins.[22] Thus, addition of small doses of prostaglandin to the treatment regimen increases the efficacy of mifepristone as an abortifacient.[4]

The combination of mifepristone and a prostaglandin is used for early abortion in France, China, the United Kingdom, and Sweden. The gestational age limit is 49 days of amenorrhea in France and China and 63 days in the United Kingdom and Sweden. The regimen used in Europe involves an initial evaluation and administration of the mifepristone followed by a return visit in about 2 days. If the woman has not aborted by this time, she is given a prostaglandin analogue and observed for 4 hours. The woman is instructed to return in about 2 weeks to confirm that the abortion has succeeded. A similar protocol will be used by practitioners in the United States once mifepristone is available.

Although mifepristone receives most of the attention, it is actually the prostaglandin that causes the abortion. How well the regimen works is more dependent on the type of

TABLE 2. Medical Abortion: Data from Clinical Trials

	Mifepristone/Misoprostol*	Methotrexate/Misoprostol†
Overall efficacy (≤ 49 days' gestation)	97%	91%
Interval between administration of each drug	2 days	5–7 days
Side effects		
Average duration of bleeding	10 days	10 days
Nausea	40%	19%
Vomiting	15%	9%
Diarrhea	10%	7%

* Data compiled from Peyron R, Aubény E, Targosz V, et al: Early termination of pregnancy with mifepristone (RU 486) and the orally active prostaglandin misoprostol. N Engl J Med 328:1509, 1993.

† Data compiled from Creinin MD, Vittinghoff E, Keder L, et al: Methotrexate and misoprostol for early abortion: A multicenter trial. I. Safety and efficacy. Contraception 53:321, 1996.

prostaglandin used in combination with the mifepristone. In the United Kingdom, for example, gemeprost is commonly used and provides effective expulsion through 63 days' gestation. An alternative prostaglandin, misoprostol, is mostly effective only through 49 days' gestation. Of the various prostaglandins studied in Europe and China in combination with mifepristone, misoprostol is the only one available in the United States and Canada. Misoprostol is an inexpensive PGE_1 analogue oral preparation that has been available in the United States since 1988. It is stable at room temperature, unlike the other prostaglandin formulations, which require refrigeration. Misoprostol is used to prevent gastric ulcers in persons taking antiinflammatory drugs on a long-term basis.

The first large-scale study using the mifepristone/misoprostol combination involved 878 women pregnant up to 49 days' gestation (Table 2).[24] The subjects were divided into two groups: 488 women received a single dose of misoprostol and 390 received the same treatment followed by a second dose of misoprostol 200 μg orally if the abortion had not occurred within 4 hours. A total of 4% of women had an abortion solely from the mifepristone, and 67% had the abortion within 4 hours of receiving the misoprostol. The success rate for women in the first group was 96.9% (95% CI 94.1–97.7%); using a second dose increased the success rate in group 2 to 98.7% (95% CI 96.8–99.5%). Uterine bleeding lasted 9 ± 4 and 10 ± 4 days in the two groups, respectively, and one woman (in group 1) required a transfusion. Approximately 80% of women had cramping, for which about 15% received a nonopiate analgesic. Nausea, vomiting, and diarrhea occurred in about 40%, 15%, and 10% of women, respectively, after the misoprostol. Thus, abortion could be accomplished with a regimen solely involving taking pills 2 days apart.

As the use of oral misoprostol with mifepristone became more common, reports began to appear in the literature about using misoprostol vaginally with fewer gastrointestinal side effects. El-Rafaey et al. reported study of 100 women using vaginal misoprostol in combination with mifepristone in 1994[13] and followed this study with a randomized trial in women pregnant up to 63 days' gestation, comparing mifepristone 600 mg followed by misoprostol 800 μg orally or vaginally (130 and and 133 subjects, respectively, per group) 48 hours later.[14] Slightly less than 3% of patients aborted from just the mifepristone, 95% aborted with the vaginal misoprostol, and 87% with oral. Moreover, 93% of the vaginal misoprostol group aborted within 4 hours, as compared with 78% of the oral group. The incidence of nausea (60% vs. 70%), vomiting (31% vs. 44%), and diarrhea (18% vs. 36%) was much lower with the vaginal than the oral misoprostol group. The higher efficacy with vaginal versus oral misoprostol in equivalent doses demonstrates the superiority of the vaginal route of administration.

Methotrexate

Because of the lack of availability of mifepristone in the United States and other countries, alternative drug regimens to effect early abortion have been developed. The most notable is the combination of methotrexate and misoprostol first described by Creinin and Darney in 1993.[8] Just as mifepristone is mislabeled as "the abortion pill," methotrexate is commonly labeled as "a cancer drug." The proper drug classification for methotrexate is an antimetabolite and, like mifepristone, it also has many uses. Methotrexate is approved by the Food and Drug Administration for use in the treatment of neoplastic diseases, rheumatoid arthritis, and psoriasis. Other common uses include the treatment of systemic lupus erythematosus, dermatomyositis, severe asthma, Crohn's disease, extrauterine pregnancy, and early abortion.

When used in the treatment of cancer, methotrexate is given in high-dose regimens. Other medical conditions for which methotrexate can be used involve low doses; this is important since toxicity is dose-dependent. High-dose versus low-dose, though, is not actually a comparison of absolute quantity administered at one time but the quantity administered over a given time (area under the curve). Thus, a single 85-mg injection of methotrexate is low-dose treatment, and a 50-mg injection 5 days in a row is a relatively high-dose treatment.

Because of its use in cancer therapies, methotrexate is falsely associated with undesirable and dangerous side effects. Specifically, high-dose methotrexate can affect the lining of the gastrointestinal tract, bone marrow, and pulmonary interstitium. With very high doses, renal toxicity and alopecia can occur. However, with low doses such as those used for abortion, side effects are usually limited to minimal gastrointestinal problems including nausea, vomiting, or diarrhea. The literature contains only isolated reports of bone marrow suppression resulting in severe leukopenia[21] and alopecia[29] in patients treated for ectopic pregnancy with the same dose of methotrexate used for abortion.

Methotrexate has been available in the United States since 1954. It does not affect the ovary or oocytes. Gonadal dysfunction after high-dose combination chemotherapy treatment regimens containing methotrexate has been reported but is felt to be unlikely due to the methotrexate and more likely the result of alkylating agents such as cyclophosphamide.[3] Seven women treated solely with high-dose methotrexate for osteosarcoma were found to have no resultant ovarian dysfunction.[25] Additionally, women treated with chemotherapy including methotrexate for gestational trophoblastic tumors have normal reproductive function in the future.[30] When methotrexate is used in a similar low-dose treatment for ectopic pregnancy, follow-up studies have demonstrated that the menses return normally and pregnancy rates are similar to those achieved by traditional surgical treatment of ectopic pregnancy.[26] Thus, methotrexate has no effect on future fertility and does not increase the risk of fetal anomalies in future pregnancies. Although fertility is unaffected, no long-term studies have addressed the theoretical possibility of decreased ovarian reserve and the potential impact on the age of menopause. However, a short-term low-dose treatment is unlikely to cause significant oocyte depletion.

The use of methotrexate for abortion stemmed from a natural progression of medical technology. Methotrexate had been used for decades as a highly effective chemotherapeutic agent against molar pregnancy and choriocarcinoma, tumors containing cancerous trophoblastic tissue. If methotrexate was effective for potentially life-threatening cancerous trophoblast, it should be effective against potentially life-threatening noncancerous trophoblast in the fallopian tube (ectopic pregnancy). From 1982–1995,

19 studies using various high-dose regimens of methotrexate with or without leucovorin rescue were published with a cumulative efficacy of 286/303 (94.4%). From 1993–1996, an additional six studies were published describing a single-dose intramuscular treatment regimen of 50 mg/m^2 with a cumulative efficacy of 238/275 (86.5%). The largest of these studies was reported by Stovall and colleagues; surgical management of the ectopic pregnancy was required in only 7 of 120 (5.8%).[27] The use of methotrexate for abortion took the final step in the natural progression since it should have similar effects on both extrauterine and intrauterine trophoblast.

Abortion with methotrexate followed by the prostaglandin misoprostol can be performed in women pregnant up to 49 days' gestation as established by vaginal ultrasound. Current published research supports the use of methotrexate in a dose of 50 mg/m^2 injected intramuscularly. The misoprostol dose (800 μg) can safely be self-administered intravaginally by the woman at home 5–7 days after the methotrexate with the same tablets used for oral dosing. The medicines are creating a miscarriage, a natural occurrence in pregnancy that women are able to safely manage themselves at home. More than 99% of the women treated in published trials had adequate pain management with self-administered oral medication. The patient returns to the office approximately 1 week after the methotrexate for a vaginal ultrasound to assess the uterine cavity. If the gestational sac is absent, the treatment is complete. If the gestational sac is still present, the misoprostol dose is repeated. If no embryonic cardiac activity is present, the patient can return in 4 weeks. If embryonic cardiac activity is present, the patient returns in 1 week. At that time, vaginal ultrasound is repeated and a suction abortion performed if embryonic cardiac activity is still present. If the gestational sac is absent, treatment is complete. If the sac is still present but no embryonic cardiac activity is present, the patient can return in 3 weeks for follow-up.

Almost all subjects who do not pass the pregnancy within 24 hours of the first or second dose of misoprostol will pass the pregnancy after a few days to a few weeks. This usually happens about 3½ weeks after methotrexate administration. During the time after misoprostol administration that the woman is waiting for the pregnancy to pass, bleeding will stop and she will not feel pregnant. Most commonly, she will have slight cramping or light bleeding a day or two before the pregnancy passes. The patient can be reassured that she will not have heavy bleeding and severe cramping without any notice. Of the patients who have to wait for the pregnancy to pass, approximately 96% will pass the pregnancy completely within 35 days after the methotrexate injection.[11]

The largest single trial using methotrexate and misoprostol conducted to date reported a series of 300 women pregnant up to 56 days' gestation treated with methotrexate 50 mg/m^2 intramuscularly followed 7 days later by misoprostol 800 μg vaginally (see Table 2).[11] The misoprostol dose was repeated 24 hours later if abortion did not occur. Overall, 88% of subjects completely aborted without the need for a surgical procedure. Because of the study size it was possible to discriminate efficacy by gestational age, with rates of 91% up to 49 days' gestation and 82% between 50 and 56 days' gestation. However, only 70% of subjects had completed the abortion by 14 days after the methotrexate. Bleeding lasted 7–10 days followed by spotting for an additional 3–5 days. Side effects occurred after both methotrexate and misoprostol administration, but some of the methotrexate side effects could simply be a result of "morning sickness." Following methotrexate, nausea occurred in 19%, vomiting in 9%, diarrhea in 7%, headache in 9%, dizziness in 4%, warmth/hot flashes in 3%, and oral ulcers in 1%. After misoprostol, nausea occurred in 12%, vomiting in 8%, diarrhea in 7%, and subjective fever/chills in 3% of patients. Preliminary work by Creinin has demonstrated that oral methotrexate 50 mg may also be effective in early abortion treatment regimens.[6]

Because methotrexate is an antimetabolite, its use in early pregnancy is a concern; if the pregnancy continues and a surgical abortion is not performed, congenital anomalies could occur. Just as important a concern is the association of misoprostol use in the first trimester with two specific anomalies. Five cases of a frontal/temporal defect in the skull without other anomalies have been described.[15] Also reported are limb abnormalities, often in association with a Möbius sequence[16] (mask-like facies with bilateral sixth and seventh nerve palsy and frequently coincident micrognathia). The women in all of these cases took misoprostol during early pregnancy in doses similar to that used for abortion with both mifepristone and methotrexate. Thus, the potential for teratogenicity is an important issue for both types of medical abortion regimens. As such, it must be emphasized to the patient before she begins a medical abortion that the agents being used to effect the abortion can cause anomalies in the ongoing pregnancy. Thus, she must be certain of her decision to have an abortion and be willing to have a surgical abortion should the medications not cause abortion.

ACCEPTABILITY OF MEDICAL ABORTION

No published studies have addressed the particular issue of acceptability of medical or surgical abortion in adolescents. Analyses of acceptability of methotrexate/misoprostol abortion demonstrated that the primary reason women in the United States wanted a medical abortion was to avoid some aspect of the surgical procedure.[7,10] In general, acceptability of medical abortion is very favorable: the experience was described as favorable 87–88% of the time in women who had a mifepristone/prostaglandin abortion[2,20] and about 90% in women who had a methotrexate/misoprostol abortion.[7,10] In Sweden, 71% of subjects questioned stated they would choose this medical method again rather than a surgical abortion.[20] The same response was cited by 80% of subjects in China.[28] Interestingly, the choice of the medical method for a future abortion was less favorable in women who had a prior surgical abortion (70%) compared with women who had not had a surgical abortion (85%). Similar results were found in two acceptability trials of methotrexate and misoprostol abortion: 81% and 83%, respectively, in women who had a prior surgical abortion and 87% and 98%, respectively, in those who had not had a surgical abortion.[7,10] This demonstrates a greater inclination of women who had never experienced a surgical abortion to be more "afraid" or "nervous" of the procedure than those who had had the procedure. This may be of particular importance when dealing with an adolescent. Work by Henshaw further demonstrates this point.[18] Among women in a research study who chose medical abortion, 95% would choose that method again. However, among women who had no preference and were randomized to receive a medical abortion, only 74% stated they would choose the medical option again. The main predictor of acceptability among these women was gestational age: 92% of women pregnant up to 49 days' gestation compared with 68% of women at 50–63 days' gestation stated they would choose the medical regimen again. Of the women randomized to vacuum aspiration, 87% stated they would choose that method again. This research supports the fact that women who desire a medical abortion are very satisfied with the results, but when the medical and surgical methods are equally available and accessible, the surgical method may be more acceptable in women at more then 49 days' gestation.

MEDICAL ABORTION BY PEDIATRICIANS

Adolescents are a unique population for medical abortion. They present the theoretical potential to not be compliant with ascribed follow-up regimens or treatment protocols. However, the literature has repeatedly shown that adolescents, when it comes to contraception and abortion, act similarly to adults. Acceptability and discontinuation rates for levonorgestrel implants are identical in adolescents and adults.[12] Similarly, women younger than 21 who are treated with methotrexate for ectopic pregnancies have similar efficacy and compliance as older women.[23]

A medical abortion is not a means to make abortion an easier decision for the adolescent who is uncertain about whether to continue the pregnancy. Once she is sure that she desires an abortion, counseling can focus on the methodologic options; this discussion needs to include the risks, benefits, and side effects of medical and surgical abortions. It is important to emphasize the necessity of follow-up and number of visits for a medical abortion. Bleeding will be much heavier than with menses (and potentially with severe cramping) and is best described as comparable to having a miscarriage. Even more important is the need to emphasize that medical abortion, whether it involves regimens with mifepristone or methotrexate, does not work as well as surgical abortion, which has a failure rate of about 1%.

My experience with medical abortion in adolescents is limited by the fact that I practice in Pennsylvania, a state that requires parental consent. As such, all of my adolescent patients are counseled and treated with the knowledge and presence of a parent. The counseling for the adolescent patient is no different from that for the adult: abortion is a personal decision that she needs to make based on her own wishes and future considerations and not those of anyone else, including her parents. As is the case for most women, teen and adult, the decision to have an abortion is usually set even before she contacts the abortion provider. Compliance and follow-up is not a greater problem with the adolescent than with the adult. In fact, the adult is usually more of a problem because her situation is not monitored; the teen with parental involvement is virtually always compliant.

The issue for the adolescent as to whether to have the abortion medically or surgically is more set by her personal beliefs, fears, and biases; again, this is no different than in an adult. Whereas a surgical abortion must occur on the weekend to avoid missing school, the medical abortion can occur any day because she can administer the misoprostol at home after school and return to school the following day. However, the teen needs to keep in mind that as many as 30% of patients will need to wait for the pregnancy to pass and that this could begin to happen at school. This potential for unpredictability needs to be balanced against the benefit of noninvasiveness and whatever other personal reasons are important. In general, teens tolerate (or do not tolerate) the bleeding and cramping as well as an adult.

Ironically, the experience of the adolescent appears to be more set by the tone of the relationship with the consenting parent rather than her own attitude. An involved parent allows for built-in support at home before, during, and after the abortion process. Parents who are very busy with work or activities outside the home usually lack the ability to provide the support needed for the procedure. This type of patient becomes obvious to the provider: the parent pulls out her work calendar to schedule appointments and calls frequently to reschedule visits because of sudden conflicts. These are also the teens who are more likely to get pregnant again because of a lack of a father in the home or a poor relationship with their mother.

Pediatricians and family practitioners should be able to provide medical abortion services as long as they are committed to understanding and providing all that is necessary for the patient. Medical abortion is a much more involved process for the practitioner than surgical abortion. Both procedures involve decision counseling and a description of the procedure, risks, and benefits. The provider needs to have a full understanding of both procedures to provide adequate counseling and compare the differences, advantages, and disadvantages to the patient. Most importantly, the provider needs to be available 24 hours a day to handle questions, provide support, and treat urgent situations that may arise, including inadequate pain control and significant hemorrhage. Because of the potential need for emergent curettage, the pediatrician or family physician must be trained to provide such services or work in conjunction with a gynecologist who can provide consultative services 24 hours a day.

Pediatricians who commit themselves to providing these services can be a valuable resource for their patients. As a primary care provider, the pediatrician has the potential to have a unique relationship with the adolescent that an abortion facility may not be able to provide. However, the pediatrician who provides medical abortion services also must be committed to providing contraceptive care and obtaining continuing education in relation to contraception and abortion. For many pediatricians, this may be more than they wish to handle as primary care providers unless they are specialists in adolescent medicine.

CONCLUSION

Medical abortion is a safe and effective alternative to surgical abortion. Primary care providers, including pediatricians for the adolescent population, can provide such services safely if they are properly trained to understand the advantages and disadvantages of medical abortion versus surgical abortion, understand the medications used and their potential side effects, and have the ability to provide emergent surgical curettage when needed. Proper patient selection for each type of abortion method is the key to ensuring patient compliance and satisfaction for both adults and adolescents.

References

1. American Academy of Pediatrics: The adolescent's right to confidential care when considering abortion. Pediatrics 97:746–751, 1996.
2. Bachelot A, Cludy L, Spira A: Conditions for choosing between drug-induced and surgical abortions. Contraception 45:546–559, 1992.
3. Bines J, Oleske DM, Cobleigh MA: Ovarian function in premenopausal women treated with adjuvant chemotherapy for breast cancer. J Clin Oncol 14:1718–1729, 1996.
4. Bygdeman M, Swahn M-L: Progesterone receptor blockage. Effect on uterine contractility and early pregnancy. Contraception 32:45–51, 1985.
5. CDC Surveillance Summaries: Abortion Surveillance—United States, 1991. MMWR 44(SS-2):23–53, 1995.
6. Creinin MD: Oral methotrexate and vaginal misoprostol for early abortion. Contraception 54:15–18, 1996.
7. Creinin MD, Burke AE: Methotrexate and misoprostol for early abortion: A multicenter trial. Acceptability. Contraception 54:19–22, 1996.
8. Creinin MD, Darney PD: Methotrexate and misoprostol for early abortion. Contraception 48:339–348, 1993.
9. Creinin MD, Edwards J: Early abortion: Surgical and medical options. Curr Probl Obstet Gynecol Fertil 20:6–32, 1997.
10. Creinin MD, Park M: Acceptability of abortion with methotrexate and misoprostol. Contraception 52:41–44, 1995.
11. Creinin MD, Vittinghoff E, Keder L, et al: Methotrexate and misoprostol for early abortion: A multicenter trial. I. Safety and efficacy. Contraception 53:321–327, 1996.
12. Cullins VE, Remsburg RE, Blumenthal PD, Huggins GR: Comparison of adolescent and adult experiences with Norplant levonorgestrel contraceptive implants. Obstet Gynecol 83:1026–1032, 1994.
13. El-Rafaey H: Early induction of abortion by a combination of oral mifepristone and misoprostol administered by the vaginal route. Contraception 49:111–114, 1994.
14. El-Rafaey H, Rajasekar D, Abdalla M, et al: Induction of abortion with mifepristone (RU 486) and oral or vaginal misoprostol. N Engl J Med 332:983–987, 1995.

15. Fonseca W, Alencar AJA, Mota FSB, Coelho HLL: Misoprostol and congenital malformations. Lancet 338:56, 1991.
16. Gonzalez CH, Vargas R, Perez AB, et al: Limb deficiency with or without Möbius sequence in seven Brazilian children associated with misoprostol use in the first trimester of pregnancy. Am J Med Genet 47:59–61, 1993.
17. Henshaw SK: The impact of requirements for parental consent on minors' abortions in Mississippi. Fam Plann Perspect 27:120–122, 1995.
18. Henshaw RC, Naji SA, Russell IT, Templeton AA: Comparison of medical abortion with surgical vacuum aspiration: Women's preferences and acceptability of treatment. BMJ 307:714–717, 1993.
19. Henshaw SK, Van Vort J: Teenage abortion, birth and pregnancy statistics. Fam Plann Perspect 21:85–88, 1989.
20. Holmgren K: Women's evaluation of three early abortion methods. Acta Obstet Gynecol Scand 71:616–623, 1992.
21. Isaacs JD Jr, McGehee RP, Cowan BD: Life-threatening neutropenia following treatment of ectopic pregnancy: A report of two cases. Obstet Gynecol 88:694–696, 1996.
22. Kelly RW, Healy DL, Cameron MJ, et al: RU 486 stimulation of $PGF_{2\alpha}$ production in isolated endometrial cells in short term culture. In Beaulieu EE, Siegel S (eds): The Antiprogestin Steroid RU 486 and Human Fertility Control. New York, Plenum, 1985, pp 259–262.
23. McCord ML, Muram D, Powell MP, Arheart KL: Methotrexate therapy for ectopic pregnancy in adolescents. J Pediatr Adolesc Gynecol 9:71–73, 1996.
24. Peyron R, Aubény E, Targosz V, et al: Early termination of pregnancy with mifepristone (RU 486) and the orally active prostaglandin misoprostol. N Engl J Med 328:1509–1513, 1993.
25. Shamberger RC, Rosenberg SA, Seipp CA, et al: Effects of high-dose methotrexate and vincristine on ovarian and testicular functions in patients undergoing postoperative adjuvant treatment of osteosarcoma. Cancer Treat Rep 65:739–746, 1981.
26. Stovall TG, Ling FW, Buster JE: Reproductive performance after methotrexate treatment of ectopic pregnancy. Am J Obstet Gynecol 162:1620–1624, 1990.
27. Stovall TG, Ling FW, Gray LA: Single-dose methotrexate for treatment of ectopic pregnancy. Obstet Gynecol 77:754–757, 1991.
28. Tang GWK, Lau OWK, Yip P: Further acceptability evaluation of RU 486 and ONO 802 as abortifacient agents in a Chinese population. Contraception 48:267–276, 1993.
29. Trout S, Kemmann E: Reversible alopecia after single-dose methotrexate treatment in a patient with ectopic pregnancy. Fertil Steril 64:866–867, 1995.
30. Walden PAM, Bagshawe KD: Reproductive performance of women successfully treated for gestational trophoblastic tumors. Am J Obstet Gynecol 125:1108–1114, 1976.

One Test Too Many: Toward an Integrated Approach to Psychosomatic Disorders

WALTER D. ROSENFELD, M.D.
GARY A. WALCO, Ph.D.

Associate Professor of Clinical Pediatrics
College of Physicians and Surgeons of Columbia University
Adolescent/Young Adult Center for Health
Morristown Memorial Hospital
Morristown, New Jersey (WDR)
and
Associate Professor of Pediatrics
University of Medicine and Dentistry
New Jersey Medical School
Chief, Section of Pediatric Psychology
Hackensack University Medical Center
Hackensack, New Jersey (GAW)

Reprint requests to:
Walter D. Rosenfeld, M.D.
Adolescent/Young Adult Center for Health
Morristown Memorial Hospital
100 Madison Avenue
Morristown, NJ 07962

Providers of health care for adolescents are all too familiar with complaints such as recurrent abdominal pain, headaches, and chest pain. Despite their frequent occurrence and discussions in medical textbooks for decades, management of these problems has been a challenge, even to the most experienced practitioner. More recently, symptoms such as chronic fatigue, arthralgias, and "total body aches" have been seen with increasing frequency in primary care practices. Experimental and empirical models for disorders such as peptic ulcer disease, inflammatory bowel disease, and pain associated with chronic illness support the notion that psychologic and somatic elements are closely and inseparably interwoven.[10] In fact, they are so closely connected that if the approach to management addresses one element to the exclusion of the other, it is likely to be met with failure.

It is apparent from the medical literature that for an array of problems, including chronic fatigue syndrome (CFS), fibromyalgia, and other disorders that typically have strong mind-body connections, there is no consensus about pathogenesis or etiology (Table 1). Even for diagnoses with extensively studied pathophysiology, such as diabetes mellitus and reactive airway disease, the impact of emotional factors on disease status is clear.

This chapter offers a rational and effective approach to disorders in which both physiologic and psychologic components are substantially involved. Chronic fatigue syndrome is used as an example of a relatively common, yet enigmatic disorder that is often frustrating for patients, parents, and physicians alike.

TABLE 1. Problems with Strong Mind-Body Connections that May Complicate Diagnosis and Management

Headache	Myofascial pain syndrome
Chest pain	Reflex sympathetic dystrophy
Irritable bowel syndrome	Vocal cord dysfunction
Recurrent abdominal pain	Reactive airway disease
Lyme disease	Diabetes mellitus
Fibromyalgia	

CASE STUDY

A 14-year-old girl, who apparently had been in good health, is brought to the pediatrician's office with a 3-month history of relentless fatigue, intermittent headache, and scattered aches and pains. Her sleep pattern has become increasingly disturbed, with difficulty falling asleep at night. No fever, weight loss, or other specific symptoms have been reported, but the current problems are not improving. The patient is beginning to miss days of school as well as social interactions with her friends. She denies feeling sad or depressed; her parents confirm that her academic performance remains good and that she remains popular among her friends. A more thorough history reveals that the patient had a moderately severe sore throat and upper respiratory illness immediately before onset of chronic symptoms. Physical examination is entirely within normal limits, except that the patient has a somewhat depressed affect. Laboratory tests, including complete blood count, sedimentation rate, Epstein-Barr virus titers, and Lyme titer, are negative.

PHYSIOLOGIC APPROACH

The scenario outlined above has become all too familiar, and chronic fatigue syndrome certainly may be the diagnosis. Further history and physical examination should focus on identifying signs and symptoms associated with other more serious diagnoses that may give persistent fatigue.[8] Examples include infectious mononucleosis, cytomegalovirus infection, hypothyroidism, anemia, diabetes mellitus, adrenocortical insufficiency, and a primary depressive disorder. In addition, for each patient cardinal symptoms often need to be investigated more thoroughly. For instance, headache with a background of allergies should prompt a consideration of chronic sinusitis. Sleep disturbance with daytime somnolence in the overweight patient may be part of a sleep apnea syndrome. Prominent joint symptoms, especially if objective findings have been observed, may be related to rheumatologic diseases such as systemic lupus erythematosus, juvenile rheumatoid arthritis, or Lyme disease.

If a thorough history and physical examination of a patient with persistent fatigue do not suggest a specific diagnosis such as inflammatory bowel disease, chronic renal failure, hypothyroidism, human immunodeficiency virus infection, or substance abuse, at least a minimal laboratory evaluation should be performed. Basic tests, such as a complete blood count (e.g, anemia, leukopenia, leukocytosis), chemistry profile (e.g., elevated liver enzymes, azotemia, hyperglycemia), sedimentation rate, thyroid function tests, and urinalysis (e.g., glycosuria, proteinuria, hematuria) may yield valuable information. When all of these tests are normal, making it reasonably clear that serious illness has been excluded, we still may feel compelled to try to document a specific cause with clear and objective findings.

Unfortunately, the specific pathophysiology of CFS remains poorly delineated. Epstein-Barr virus infection,[9] immunologic abnormalities,[1] and neurally mediated hypotension[3] are among the disorders that have been or are currently under discussion as causally related to CFS. However, even without an understanding of a specific cause (which may give rise to a specific diagnostic test), an effective approach to diagnosis and treatment is certainly needed. To aid in the collection of consistent data about clinical spectrum and prevalence, the Centers for Disease Control and Prevention (CDC) established criteria for defining CFS.[12] Although such guidelines are essential for research purposes, they are of more limited value to clinicians who need to deal with a wide array of clinical presentations, including a substantial number of patients who do not fully meet the required criteria. Thus, the clinician is left with a clinical diagnosis that cannot be substantiated with definitive, objective findings.

The situation is complicated by the fact that the patient's symptoms, often severe and relentless, are inconsistent with the objective findings. An obvious concern is that symptoms may represent depression, anxiety, or less common disorders, such as hypochondriasis or malingering. Unfortunately, if questions about psychosocial issues are introduced only after negative findings are documented, the patient and family often become frustrated and indignant, surmising that the doctor does not believe that the symptoms are "real."

PSYCHOLOGIC APPROACH

At first glance, it seems logical to focus on psychosomatic disorders from a purely psychologic perspective. This approach to chronic fatigue syndrome has a great deal of appeal. Chronic fatigue syndrome shares many diagnostic features of mood disorders (depression, dysthymia), including sleep problems, fatigue, and loss of energy. Thus, it has been speculated that CFS may be a manifestation of underlying psychiatric syndromes.[2] Kruesi et al.[11] studied adult patients with CFS and found that 75% fulfilled diagnostic criteria for various psychiatric syndromes, including depression. Others have found similar results in populations of children.[6,14]

Some features of hypochondriasis overlap with those of CFS. The cornerstone of the diagnosis of hypochondriasis is preoccupation with the notion that one has a serious disease based on the misinterpretation of bodily symptoms. This preoccupation persists despite appropriate medical evaluation and reassurance and may cause clinically significant distress or impairment in important areas of functioning. Clinical and research experience have demonstrated that adolescents with CFS are acutely occupied with physical symptoms.[4]

Research data indicate that pediatric patients with CFS resemble neither psychiatrically referred patients nor healthy peers. Carter et al.[4] administered a battery of psychologic instruments to children and adolescents with CFS and matched groups of healthy and depressed subjects. Patients with CFS were more likely to report sleepiness, sleep disturbance, low energy, decreased appetite, and reduced personal efficacy, as well as loss of pleasure in usual activities, loneliness and social isolation, mild-to-moderate feelings of unhappiness, and self-dissatisfaction than healthy peers. Patients with CFS reported more somatic complaints (headache, arthralgia, sore throat, myalgia, nausea, dizziness) than patients with depression, whereas patients with depression reported higher levels of suicidal ideation and previous suicidal behavior as well as more social isolation and ostracism. In addition, patients with CFS reported greater levels of fatigue, sleepiness, and tiredness. The authors concluded that children with CFS are not depressed in the conventional sense but are more distressed than healthy peers. Patients with CFS are less likely than depressed patients to see a role for psychologic issues in their condition and more likely to deny that they are in need of assistance.

Even when suspicion of psychologic dysfunction is high, directly confronting patients and families with the notion that the presenting symptoms are psychiatrically based is rarely productive. It is likely that the same psychologic defenses and coping mechanisms that potentiate or maintain the symptoms will become more rigid if a confrontational approach is taken. Furthermore, the likelihood that the family will accept referral to a mental health specialist under these circumstances is reduced.[13] Even if one accepts the premise that depressive disorders and CFS overlap significantly, this premise does not necessarily provide a clear pathway for treatment. In a review of the literature, Gruber et al.[7] described few controlled studies in which psychotropic medications were found helpful in CFS. The cited studies concluded that, although various agents have been noted to affect CFS symptoms positively, as a rule the response is partial and inconsistent.

TOWARD A SYNTHESIS

For many years, Western medicine has followed the dualistic perspective of René Descartes, resulting in a conceptual approach that fosters a strong dichotomy between physiologic and psychologic factors. Thus, symptoms are evaluated first to identify the pathophysiology of the condition; if it is discovered, the situation is remediated. If multiple assessments, laboratory studies, and diagnostic procedures fail to indicate a clear etiology, or if the symptoms are exaggerated compared with the known pathologic condition, it is presumed that psychologic factors are at work. Thus, only after known physiologic factors are excluded is the patient sent for psychologic or psychiatric assessment. Of course, even if the psychologic factors are salient, the repeated intensive physical evaluations by various medical subspecialists only reinforce the psychologic mechanisms that are at work. This ultimately makes the referral to a mental health practitioner more difficult.

One obvious solution is to include a psychosocial assessment at the beginning of the evaluation. Thus, the dichotomy is minimized. In addition, we are foolish to separate "physiologic" from "psychologic" factors because they appear to be flip sides of the same coin. For many years, it has been recognized that stress has a deleterious effect on gastrointestinal functioning. In the case of peptic ulcers, for example, we know that with increased stress comes sympathetic nervous system arousal, which includes increased production of gastric acids, and risk of ulceration. Is this a psychologic or physiologic phenomenon? Clearly it is both.

Furthermore, is it reasonable to assume that a syndrome is psychologically based simply because we lack the technology to identify specific physiologic mechanisms? For example, most cases of dysmenorrhea were commonly regarded as a psychologic phenomenon until the role of prostaglandins was delineated. As the specific cascade of physiologic events was demonstrated, the etiologic role of psychologic factors diminished.

Finally, recent data indicate that there may be no real distinction between "physiologic" and "psychologic" factors. In discussing inflammatory bowel disease, Mayer described the relationship among environmental stressors, acute visceral stimulation, tissue inflammation, and disruption of the hypothalamic-pituitary-adrenal (HPA) feedback loop.[10] Thus, one can comprehend the link between "psychologic" factors (stress) and "physiologic" factors (bowel inflammation). It truly becomes an impossible intellectual challenge to discern a division between the two. Indeed, in a study specifically focusing on HPA activity, significant differences were found between patients with CFS and normal subjects.[5]

Although the clinical relevance of the relationship between central nervous system activity and symptoms in psychosomatic syndromes is not in our immediate grasp, the available evidence makes it clear that it is shortsighted to maintain the dichotomous perspective that has pervaded our thinking for so many years. The ultimate goal is to have a singular, integrated approach. At this juncture, diagnostic and therapeutic endeavors must include simultaneous and parallel application of physiologic and psychologic variables. This can best be accomplished by eliciting psychosocial information from patients and families during the medical history and applying a team approach to patient care. In addition to team members focused primarily on the physiologic issues (e.g., pediatrician, adolescent medicine physician, family physician), a psychologist, psychiatrist, social worker, or other mental health professional should be an early and active participant in the care of patients with these more complex disorders. Of course, all members of the team need to have an understanding of, and appreciation for, this unified model.

References

1. Barker E, Fujimura SF, Fadem M, et al: Immunologic abnormalities associated with chronic fatigue syndrome. Clin Infect Dis 18:S136–S141, 1994.
2. Bonner D, Ron M, Chalder T: Chronic fatigue syndrome: A follow up study. J Neurol Neurosurg Psychiatry 57:617–621, 1994.
3. Bou-Holaigah I, Rowe PC, Kan J, et al: The relationship between neurally mediated hypotension and the chronic fatigue syndrome. JAMA 274:961–967, 1995.
4. Carter BD, Kronenberger WG, Edwards JF: Differential diagnosis of chronic fatigue in children: Behavioral and emotional dimensions. Develop Behav Pediatr 17:16–21, 1996.
5. Demitrack MA, Kale JK, Straus SE: Evidence for impaired activation of the hypothalamic-pituitary-adrenal axis in patients with chronic fatigue syndrome. J Clin Endocrinol Metab 73:1224–1234, 1991.
6. Garralda ME: Severe chronic fatigue syndrome in childhood: A discussion of psychopathological mechanisms. Eur Child Adolesc Psychiatry 1:111–118, 1992.
7. Gruber AJ, Hudson JI, Pope HG, et al: The management of treatment-resistant depression in disorders on the interface of psychiatry and medicine. Psychiatr Clin North Am 19:351–368, 1996.
8. Krilov LR: Chronic fatigue syndrome. Pediatr Ann 24:290–294, 1995.
9. Mawle AC, Reyes M, Schmid DS: Is chronic fatigue syndrome an infectious disease? Infect Agents Dis 2:333–341, 1994.
10. Mayer EA: Breaking down the functional and organic paradigm. Curr Opin Gastroenterol 12:3–7, 1996.
11. Kruesi MJP, Dale J, Straus SE: Psychiatric diagnoses in patients who have chronic fatigue syndrome. J Clin Psychiatry 50:53–56, 1989.
12. Reyes M, Gary HE, Dobbins JG: Surveillance for chronic fatigue syndrome—four U.S. cities, September 1989 through August 1993. MMWR 46:2–13, 1997.
13. Speckens AEM, van Hemert AM, Bolk JH: The acceptability of psychological treatment in patients with medically unexplained physical symptoms. J Psychosom Res 39:855–863, 1995.
14. Walford GA, Nelson W, McCluskey DR: Fatigue, depression, and social adjustment in chronic fatigue syndrome. Arch Dis Child 68:384–388, 1993.

Controversies in the Diagnosis and Treatment of Attention Deficit/Hyperactivity Disorder in Adolescents

ESTHER H. WENDER, M.D.

Clinical Professor of Pediatrics
Albert Einstein College of Medicine
Bronx, New York

Reprint requests to:
Esther H. Wender, M.D.
104 Ridgewood Terrace
Chappaqua, NY 10514

Attention deficit/hyperactivity disorder (AD/HD) is recognized as the most common significant behavior-problem syndrome in childhood. Over the past 10 years, it has been widely acknowledged that the syndrome persists into adolescence in about 80% of the cases recognized initially during childhood.

Despite general recognition of AD/HD as a condition that affects children and adolescents, the disorder, its diagnosis, and its treatment remain controversial. This chapter discusses general controversies, particularly those that apply to AD/HD in adolescence.

GENERAL CONTROVERSIES

Is AD/HD a Disorder?

The concept of a syndrome as a disorder seems to require the presence of an underlying pathology to account for not only the classic symptoms but also some of the variability in manifestations of the syndrome. Using this gauge, AD/HD cannot be called a disorder. A possible underlying pathology has been identified in only a handful of cases.[2,11] Most investigators acknowledge that many pathologic mechanisms are likely to account for the syndrome, that underlying biologic phenomena will explain only a portion of the symptomatology, and that the impact of environmental factors may range from minimal to extensive. It is also clear that, even if some pathologic precursors are identified, the severity of problems varies along a continuum and a threshold for diagnosis will always be an issue, much as it is for hypertension, in which an arbitrary cut-off level of elevated blood pressure is established based on the likelihood that related problems will develop as a result of that elevation. When diagnoses are based on findings that occur along a continuum, patients may qualify for the diagnosis at one point and then not qualify at another. Such variability in diagnosis over time is not consistent with most peoples' concept of "disorder."

How should AD/HD be characterized if not as a disorder? This author prefers to think of it as a syndrome consisting of extremes of temperament. Even though the severity of symptoms is variable and no biologic marker can be found to diagnose the condition independently, the syndrome cannot be ignored; there is considerable evidence that serious problems result from the condition. Also, although an underlying pathology cannot be identified in most cases, there is ample circumstantial evidence that some type of biologic mechanism is responsible for AD/HD. This circumstantial evidence consists of research findings indicating a genetic contribution to the syndrome in most cases. In the treatment of AD/HD, the clinician should acknowledge the underlying biologic contribution because adults who encounter AD/HD commonly blame the child for failure to behave properly. Children and adolescents and the important adults in their lives can respond more appropriately to this syndrome when issues of blame are removed.

Labeling of AD/HD and Treatment

For professionals who have diagnosed and treated AD/HD for many years, the concern is that too few of the affected children and adolescents are being recognized and treated. The prevalence of AD/HD in childhood ranges from 3–10% of elementary school-aged children, with the higher figures applying to a lower socioeconomic population. Despite the dramatic increase in the number of children identified and treated with stimulant medication over the past 6 years, clinical experience is that many cases of AD/HD remain unrecognized and untreated. Two studies that examined the increase in prescriptions for methylphenidate (Ritalin) in comparison with the expected number of children and adolescents with AD/HD found that the number treated remains less, and often much less, than the number expected from prevalence calculations.[7,9] In a study by Safer et al., the increase in the amount of prescribed Ritalin could be accounted for, in part, by the number of children who continue to be treated into adolescence,[9] which represents an appropriate change in clinical practice.

Public awareness of AD/HD and clinical practices associated with the syndrome have increased significantly, perhaps as a result of (1) greater media attention arising from the critical mass of recognized and treated patients, (2) the impact of the national family support group called Children with Attention Deficit Disorder, and (3) the increased amount of training of physicians, psychologists, and teachers regarding the effects of this syndrome.

Has there been a real increase in AD/HD in the population? Over the past 20 years, the period during which appropriate prevalence studies have been conducted, there has been no dramatic change in prevalence figures. An increasing number of prevalence studies are being conducted in different countries with different cultures, and, despite some variability in prevalence, the syndrome is recognized in a significant percentage of school-aged children in all cultures where it has been studied.

CONTROVERSIES IN ADOLESCENTS

Diagnosis of AD/HD Behaviors

The diagnosis of AD/HD behaviors is an issue that confronts the clinician dealing with this syndrome in children of all ages, because the diagnosis of the "disorder" is based almost entirely on a history of the defining behaviors obtained from parents and others who observe an affected child or adolescent frequently. The behaviors that characterize AD/HD are seen in "normal" children and adolescents and should be considered a problem, and thus positive evidence of AD/HD, only when they occur more frequently or at a greater level of severity than is normal for the person's developmental age. Therefore, how does the clinician decide if the behavior is normal or abnormal? A number of clinical guidelines may help. Parents and teachers should be asked to compare the adolescent's behavior to that of others of the same age or in the same classroom. Questionnaires designed to help in the diagnostic process always incorporate a severity scale that requires the respondent to rate the adolescent's behavior in comparison with that of others of the same age. In the final analysis, however, the decision about whether the behavior is normal or abnormal is based on responses of the informants and the clinician's judgment regarding the accuracy and objectivity of the observers.

Evolution of AD/HD in Adolescents

Clinicians who have followed children with AD/HD into adolescence have learned that many of the problems persist into the teenage years and that new problems also frequently develop. Adolescents who were diagnosed with AD/HD in childhood continue to meet diagnostic criteria for AD/HD in adolescence in about 40% of cases. An additional 40% of adolescents with childhood-diagnosed AD/HD no longer meet standardized criteria for AD/HD but continue to display some of the symptomatology, and many of these adolescents qualify for other, related diagnoses,[4] including conduct disorders, anxiety disorders, mood disorders such as dysthymia, and a variety of academic problems. As adolescents, children with AD/HD often become significant underachievers, and they have much higher than expected rates of school dropout, suspensions, and expulsions. This increased impact on academic performance leads to another controversy in the field of AD/HD: whether AD/HD is a learning disability or purely a behavioral syndrome.

AD/HD: A Learning Disability or Behavior Syndrome?

Although younger children with AD/HD have attention deficits, the deficits are usually manifested by behaviors such as moving from one activity to another or "not listening" to requests or instructions. However, during adolescence, a time when school work becomes more complex, attention deficits begin to have a direct impact on academic performance. For example, the junior or senior high school student may experience great difficulty completing long-term assignments that involve a number of steps, such as gathering information, organizing that information, and presenting it in written or oral format. Adolescents with AD/HD also may have great difficulty studying for tests, a process that begins with daily lectures or reading assignments and is followed by a review of all of the accumulated information. Adolescents with persistent AD/HD symptoms may do reasonably well with daily assignments but have great difficulty organizing and retaining the information for examination. These are examples of *learning problems* that may be based primarily on AD/HD behaviors. Additional academic problems are clearly due to the *behavioral* issues of AD/HD. Adolescents with AD/HD, for example, demonstrate increasing problems with completing assigned work. They may become disruptive in the classroom and are more likely to be suspended or expelled for behavioral infractions. Therefore, whether the significant academic problems of the adolescent with AD/HD are due to behavioral problems or a specific type of AD/HD-related learning disability is not clear.

The Relationship between AD/HD and Conduct Disorder

Another controversy centers on what are described as *conduct problems* during adolescence and their relationship to AD/HD in childhood. A significant number of children with AD/HD develop conduct problems in adolescence and may qualify for the diagnosis of conduct disorder.[6,10] Such problems include (1) abuse of alcohol or drugs, (2) excessive arrests for infractions such as larceny or arson, (3) excessive aggressiveness in the form of fighting, and (4) sexual promiscuity and aggression such as rape. Prospective studies suggest that children with AD/HD who also have oppositional-defiant disorder (ODD) are much more likely to manifest conduct problems during adolescence. The percentage of children with AD/HD who also manifest ODD behaviors ranges from 30–50%—so there continues to be a substantial population of AD/HD children who are at high risk for these more severe adolescent behavior problems. The association between childhood AD/HD and adolescent conduct problems is so strong that all adolescents presenting with conduct problems such as those mentioned above should be evaluated for the possibility of childhood AD/HD, especially since AD/HD still is frequently overlooked.

According to most studies, conduct problems in adolescence are particularly difficult to treat.[8] However, a connection to an earlier history of AD/HD may lead to different approaches to therapy, such as medication, which may be especially helpful. Clinicians, however, often have difficulty shifting from a focus on conduct problems as a social issue to a focus on the possible contribution of a biologically based childhood disorder. It may be especially difficult to obtain relevant history for adolescents whose conduct problems have led to placement in foster homes or detention facilities, thus eliminating the primary observers of childhood behavior. In addition, many adolescents with conduct problems come from dysfunctional families, and it may be difficult to separate family dysfunction from the symptoms that characterize AD/HD. However, the clinician should attempt this differential diagnosis because an earlier history of AD/HD potentially has a positive impact on treatment options.

Treatment in Adolescents Versus Children

The treatment of AD/HD throughout the child/adolescent age span remains controversial. A growing number of studies, however, demonstrate that stimulant medication is the single best treatment. Psychological therapies have been shown to be helpful only in combination with medication.[3]

An important question is whether stimulant medication is helpful in adolescents. At least 50% of adolescents who continue to manifest AD/HD symptomatology but 60–80% of elementary school-aged children respond favorably to stimulant medication.[5] Whether this difference is due to less accurate diagnoses in adolescence or due to a change in response to medication as a result of neurologic maturation is unknown.

However, a 50% favorable response is certainly sufficient to warrant a trial of stimulant medication, especially in adolescents with conduct problems, because this is such a serious disorder. Stimulants are known to affect favorably some of the oppositional-defiant symptoms, such as excessive temper outbursts and poor compliance with requests, that are thought to precede conduct problems.

Although short-term studies show that stimulant medication is the most effective single treatment for AD/HD at any age, long-term studies fail to demonstrate a favorable effect of medication on ultimate outcome. Thus, other approaches to treatment continue to be an important issue. One unanswered question is whether adolescents respond in special ways to psychotherapeutic approaches to treatment. Many clinicians describe favorable responses to psychotherapy during adolescence, when the ability to evaluate self in relation to others improves. Behavior therapy approaches also have been advocated.[1] However, very few studies address psychotherapy for AD/HD in adolescence, and the studies that address psychotherapy for conduct problems are particularly negative.

CONCLUSION

Although it is generally accepted that the syndrome known as AD/HD persists into adolescence in most of the affected children, many controversial issues remain surrounding AD/HD in general and regarding the outcomes of AD/HD in adolescence and adulthood. The most significant issue involves the relationship between AD/HD in childhood and conduct disorder in adolescents and adults. Much research remains to be done.

Reference

1. Ajibola O, Clement PW: Differential effects of methylphenidate and self-reinforcement on attention deficit hyperactivity disorder. Behav Modif 19:211–213, 1995.
2. Ernst M, et al: Reduced brain metabolism in hyperactive girls. J Am Acad Child Adolesc Psychiatry 33:858, 1994.
3. Gittelman-Klein R, Abikoff H, Pollack E, et al: A controlled trial of behavior modification and methylphenidate in hyperactive children. In Whalen CK, Henker B (eds): Hyperactive Children: The Social Ecology of Identification and Treatment. New York, Academic Press, 1989, pp 221–243.
4. Gittelman R, Mannuza S, Shenker R, et al: Hyperactive boys almost grown up. Arch Gen Psychiatry 42:937–947, 1985.
5. Klorman R, Brumaghim JT, Fitzpatrick PA, et al: Clinical effects of a controlled trial of methylphenidate on adolescents with attention deficit disorder. J Am Acad Child Adolesc Psychiatry 29:702–709, 1990.
6. MacDonald VM, Achenbach TM: Attention problems versus conduct problems as six-year predictors of problem scores in a national sample. J Am Acad Child Adolesc Psychiatry 35:1237–1246, 1996.
7. Rappley MD, Gardiner JC, Jetton JR, et al: The use of methylphenidate in Michigan. Arch Pediatr Adolesc Med 149:675–679, 1995.
8. Robins LN, Price RK: Adult disorders predicted by childhood conduct problems: Results from the NIMH Epidemiologic Catchment Area Project. Psychiatry 54:116–132, 1991.
9. Safer DJ, Zito JM, Fine EM: Increased methylphenidate usage for attention deficit disorder in the 1990s. Pediatrics 98:1084–1088, 1996.
10. Taylor E, Chadwick O, Heptinstall E, et al: Hyperactivity and conduct problems as risk factors for adolescent development. J Am Acad Child Adolesc Psychiatry 35:1213–1226, 1996.
11. Zametkin AJ, Nordahl TE, Gross M, et al: Cerebral glucose metabolism in adults with hyperactivity of childhood onset. N Engl J Med 153:1361–1366, 1990.

Rebellious Adolescents: Is Toughlove the Answer?

CAROL FORD ARKIN, Ph.D.
JEFFREY B. GILLMAN, Ph.D.

Department of Psychology
Columbus Children's Hospital
Columbus, Ohio

Reprint requests to:
Carol Ford Arkin, Ph.D.
Department of Psychology
Columbus Children's Hospital
700 Children's Drive
Columbus, OH 43205

Concern about rebellious, destructive, antisocial behaviors by adolescents is prevalent among professionals and the general population. This concern is borne out by a variety of indicators that attest to the clinical and social significance of externalizing behavioral problems. Aggressiveness, conduct problems, and antisocial behaviors, for example, account for a third to half of all child and adolescent clinic referrals; moreover, patterns of disruptive behavior tend to be stable over time.[3] Some investigators have noted, in fact, that the stability of childhood aggression rivals the stability of intellectual capacity.[10] Others have argued that so many young people engage in some antisocial behaviors during adolescence that the behaviors can be considered statistically normative for this age group.[8] Overall, in terms of financial and social costs to society, disruptive behaviors are among the most costly mental disorders.[3]

Interventions for externalizing disorders offered by mental health professionals have run the gamut from individual psychotherapy, to family-based treatments, to residential programs, to community-based programs.[3] Data on help-seeking in general, however, suggest that many families who are experiencing disruptive behavior problems will turn to informal sources of help rather than to professionals.[12] Others may seek informal support while using professional services or after completing or leaving a treatment program.

Although sometimes controversial, grassroots, mutual-help groups provide one alternative, or adjunct, to professional interventions for many families. This chapter examines one example of this type of approach for externalizing behavior problems: the

Toughlove mutual-help program created by the Toughlove organization to help parents combat serious disruptive behavior problems in their children.[13]

The Toughlove program is distinguished from the term *tough love*, which has become a familiar part of everyday language and by itself can convey an emphasis on very strict discipline that is not necessarily representative of the principles and strategies used in the Toughlove program. This distinction is particularly important given that harsh discipline practices are associated with the occurrence, not amelioration, of disruptive behavior problems.

EXTERNALIZING BEHAVIOR PROBLEMS

Externalizing behavior problems in adolescents refer to an array of disruptive behaviors that include conduct problems, noncompliance, aggressiveness, antisocial behavior, impulsivity, attentional problems, or hyperactivity. The *Diagnostic and Statistical Manual of Mental Disorders, Fourth Edition* delineates three types of externalizing problems under the general heading of attention-deficit and disruptive behavior disorders: attention deficit/hyperactivity disorder (ADHD), conduct disorder (CD), and oppositional defiant disorder (ODD).[1] Research on disruptive behavior disorders clearly supports the view that they are different syndromes but have high rates of comorbidity.[7]

A number of excellent and detailed discussions of the diagnosis, developmental course, and treatment of externalizing disorders are available.[3,7,8,10] In general, the study of childhood psychopathology is a relatively new field, within which adolescents have received less attention than younger children.[4] But probably no area within childhood psychopathology has received more attention than externalizing disorders. Our understanding of disruptive behaviors has seen rapid and ongoing growth in the last three decades, particularly in terms of assessment and treatment.

In terms of treatment, family-based interventions for preadolescents, rooted in behavioral principles, presently have the best-documented results for treating conduct problems.[7] The combined use of behavior therapy and stimulant medication appears promising for the treatment of ADHD.[11]

Although behavioral interventions have been successful, positive treatment outcomes with adolescents have been the most elusive.[7] Other factors that bode poorly for successful treatment include comorbidity of disruptive behavior patterns and the presence of covert behaviors such as stealing.[7] Finally, so-called early-starters, children who begin a pattern of disruptive behavior in their early school-age years or earlier, clearly have the worst prognosis.[8,10] The stability of externalizing behaviors for children who begin this pattern early, in fact, has led a number of prominent investigators to propose conceptualizing conduct disorders as a "chronic disease"[3] and as "life-course persistent."[8]

THE TOUGHLOVE PROGRAM

In the popular 1982 book *Toughlove*, authors Phyllis and David York describe how desperation with their adolescent daughter's behavior and frustration with professional interventions led them to develop their own approach. They enlisted help from friends and established firm consequences for unacceptable behavior, a process they labeled "taking a stand." The Yorks subsequently formed Toughlove International, a nonprofit organization that sponsors and provides technical assistance to local parent-run mutual help groups. They have reported reaching more than 350,000 participants through local chapters since they began in 1978.[5]

"Taking a stand" is one of the central tenets of Toughlove. The program is rooted in the assumptions that contemporary culture is central to the origins and maintenance of adolescents' behavioral problems and that children shape their parents' behavior just as parents attempt to influence and shape their children's behavior. The Yorks argued that both of these factors contribute to parental "helplessness" and that professional counselors often increase parents' helplessness by focusing on finding underlying causes for disruptive behavior. The Toughlove approach is characterized by 10 principles for parents, which emphasize accepting their own faults, frailties, and limitations; taking action in response to problem behavior rather than focusing on understanding underlying or historic causes; and seeking the help, support, and involvement of as much of the community as possible. There is a structured format for support group meetings that includes small group problem-solving, discussion of participants' short- and long-term goals for their children's behavior, and participants' sharing of success stories.

Anecdotal evidence of Toughlove's success has been provided by the Yorks and others.[9,13,14] As is common for grassroots, mutual-help programs, however, almost no scientific data are available. In searching for evaluation of the results of the program, we were able to find one empirical study that provided descriptive information about a sample of Toughlove members.[5] This report also described the process of the support group meeting and preliminary findings regarding behavioral outcomes.

Klug sent questionnaires to 110 parents who indicated a willingness to participate in his research when recruited at regional and national Toughlove workshops. Seventy-five parents from eight states returned the questionnaires. Most of the respondents were women (80%), 40–48 years old (58%), and married (69%). Almost half of the sample attended some college, and almost a fifth had done graduate work. Mean household income was $48,400. Half the subjects described themselves as politically moderate, and about a quarter reported having conservative or liberal outlooks. Approximately two-thirds of the respondents were Catholic or Protestant, and 14% were Jewish. Of the 26% who indicated no religious affiliation, three-fourths reported they had been raised as Catholics.

A third of the subjects reported that during their childhood one or both their parents were addicted to alcohol or drugs; 15% reported that they had been addicted to substances at some time before they joined Toughlove. About 82% reported having been in therapy before joining Toughlove, and 72% had been in therapy since joining. One fifth of the respondents who had been in therapy quit after joining Toughlove.

Klug also gathered observational data from meetings of six small Toughlove support groups. Three judges coded transcripts of meetings for the frequency of occurrence of a set of "process variables" derived from reviews of the literature on mutual-help groups and on Toughlove and from informal interviews with members. Out of the six process variables examined, empathy (including emotional support and a sense of community) and assertiveness training (including informational support) accounted for 43% and 40%, respectively, of the coded behaviors in the meetings.

Finally, Klug was interested in the impact of parents' participation in Toughlove on their children's behavior problems. Parents were asked to complete a survey of their child's behavior before and after they joined Toughlove. Only half of the parents surveyed returned these questionnaires, and many of the behaviors on the survey were reported too infrequently for analysis. The data revealed reports of significant changes in nine antisocial behaviors; 85% of the changed behaviors were improved and 10% had worsened.

Overall, the only direct evaluation data we could find is positive, but it clearly is limited by the select sample and the nature of the data. Retrospective self-report data on behavioral change from only half of a select sample provides only a very rough, unsubstantiated, and preliminary indication of the actual impact of the program.

Given the paucity of direct data, an alternative means of evaluating Toughlove, although clearly speculative, is to extrapolate from what is known about the developmental course, correlates, and professional interventions for externalizing behavior problems. Although the tone of Toughlove's literature is polemic and often explicitly opposed to professional theory, elements of the program appear to be consistent with aspects of scientifically based and evaluated professional interventions.

Compatible Features of Toughlove and Scientific Literature

CONCEPTUAL SIMILARITIES

The Toughlove program was developed to counteract parental helplessness in the face of their children's severe problem behavior. Consistent with this formulation, inconsistent parental discipline, underinvolvement, and poor monitoring and supervision of the child are well-documented behaviors in families of children with externalizing behavior problems.[10] Toughlove's literature, however, emphasizes that parents are not to blame for their children's misbehavior and points to contemporary culture as causing parental helplessness. In contrast, social scientists have pointed to the causal role of poor parenting practices in the development of behavioral problems and have presented a more complex picture of the determinants of parental behavior.[10] Nevertheless, although arriving at similar conclusions by different routes, there is commonality in the importance given to inadequate and ineffective parenting.

In addition, the Toughlove program emphasizes the reciprocal influence parents and children exert on one another. Over the last three decades, recognition of reciprocal parent-child influences has grown dramatically in the developmental and clinical literatures. It is the basis of one of the most influential theoretical perspectives on antisocial behavior in children: Patterson's coercion theory.[10] Again, however, the overlap between the Toughlove philosophy and the scientific literature on this point is not absolute. Toughlove's publications strongly emphasize children's effects on parents, at times with a tone that some readers might find somewhat harsh or blaming of the children (despite their general exhortation against blaming), while they explicitly deemphasize parents' causative role in their children's behavior. The growing recognition among professionals of reciprocal causality between parents and children has expanded rather than replaced their focus on the effects that parents have on their children.

Finally, the message that "it's OK to fail" and encouragement to focus on renewed effort rather than self-blame is a consistent theme in Toughlove's literature. Conceptually, this message appears compatible with work in the area of habit change and relapse prevention, indicating that an individual's understanding of and reactions to a lapse largely determine whether it will lead to a complete reversion to old habits.[6]

CHANGE MECHANISMS

A number of aspects of the change process advocated in the Toughlove program share common features with professional interventions, particularly those rooted in behavioral principles. Consistent with their underlying emphasis on inadequate and ineffective parenting practices, both approaches emphasize effecting changes in parents' behavior as the primary route to reducing or eliminating behavior problems in their children. The Toughlove approach encourages parents to focus their efforts at change on developing explicit limits and boundaries for children and, also, on establishing and following through with consequences for misbehavior. Increased parental monitoring and contingent responses are also central, empirically supported aspects of behavior management programs.[2,10]

In addition, Toughlove's emphasis on involving as much of the community as possible is consistent with a growing emphasis in behavior programs on effecting changes across multiple systems.[37]

OTHER RELEVANT FEATURES

Parental stress, depression, and isolation have been associated with externalizing behavioral problems in children.[3,7] The social support provided by Toughlove groups may alleviate these factors for some parents. Moreover, the affiliative component, in conjunction with social demands to change parenting practices, may be able to counteract some of the negativity reported in response to therapist's (i.e., authoritative) demands to change in professional interventions.[2]

Problems and Limitations

As noted earlier, specific types of disruptive behavior disorders appear to be best understood as separate but highly overlapping conditions.[7] In addition, externalizing behavioral problems have been associated with a host of other difficulties, including learning problems, parental psychopathology, and marital conflict.[3] Treatment of co-occurring problems is likely to require a mixture of interventions tailored to the specific presenting problems. The most promising research-based treatments for ADHD and CD, for example, are a mixture of overlapping but also unique components (e.g., the use of stimulant medication to treat ADHD). The Toughlove program, however, purports to address a wide range of problem behaviors.

In addition, it is possible that families who use Toughlove as an alternative rather than as an adjunct to professional assistance run the risk that the other group members might not recognize or know how to help find treatment for concurrent problems not addressed by the group. In a related vein, children who display antisocial behaviors are also likely to lack prosocial skills.[10] Although the Toughlove program provides strategies for decreasing problem behavior, the needed adjunct of increasing positive behavior does not appear to be addressed. Moreover, it is possible that the Toughlove theme that parents are not responsible for their children's behavior inadvertently discourages parents from attending to and helping their children develop positive, prosocial behaviors.

Another limitation stems from the focus in Toughlove's literature on parental helplessness, which is only one of several types of problematic discipline associated with externalizing disorders. Other inadequate discipline styles identified by Chamberlain and Patterson, for example, include irritable-explosive discipline and inflexible-rigid discipline.[2]

Finally, Toughlove's literature appears to emphasize adolescent behavior problems occurring without warning in apparently well-adjusted children and families. It is possible that this characterization may have the greatest appeal to families of children who display an adolescent-onset pattern of antisocial behavior.[8] Also called "late-starters," these children have the best prognosis, presumably because they have a briefer history of problems and therefore more prosocial skills and less disrupted families. Speculation that Toughlove may appeal to a select population does not indicate that it is not useful in some cases, but it does highlight the value of controlled evaluation studies and the limitations in generalizing from anecdotal data.

CONCLUSIONS

In the two decades since Toughlove began, the scientific study of externalizing behavioral disorders has grown at a rapid pace. Research on treatment has established a solid base of support for family-based, behaviorally oriented interventions. The evidence at present is stronger, however, for younger children than for adolescents. Unfortunately, in the absence of direct data, it is possible only to speculate about the effectiveness of the grassroots mutual-help alternative offered in the Toughlove approach. A number of features of the program appear compatible with our current understanding of disruptive behavior disorders, and many families clearly are in need of alternatives and social support. Other features, however, raise cautions and probable limitations of the benefits of this approach, suggesting that the interventions may be inadequate for the needs of many families experiencing disruptive behavioral problems.

References

1. American Psychiatric Association: Diagnostic and Statistical Manual of Mental Disorders, 4th ed. Washington, D.C., APA, 1994.
2. Chamberlain P, Patterson GR: Discipline and child compliance in parenting. In Bornstein MH (ed): Handbook of Parenting, Vol. 4. Mahay, NJ, Lawrence Erlbaum Associates, 1995, pp 205–225.
3. Kazdin AE: Treatment of antisocial behavior in children: Current status and future directions. Psychol Bull 102:187, 1987.
4. Kazdin AE: Adolescent mental health: Prevention and treatment programs. Am Psychol 48:127, 1993.
5. Klug W: A preliminary investigation of Toughlove: Assertiveness and support in a parents' self-help group. Presented at the 98th annual meeting of the American Psychological Association, Boston, August 10–14, 1990.
6. Marlatt AG, Gordon JR (eds): Relapse Prevention. New York, Guilford Press, 1985.
7. McMahon RJ: Diagnosis, assessment, and treatment of externalizing problems in children: The role of longitudinal data. J Consult Clin Psychol 2:901, 1994.
8. Moffitt TE: Adolescence-limited and life-course-persistent antisocial behavior: A developmental taxonomy. Psychol Rev 100:674, 1993.
9. Ooms T, Owen T: Parents' role in teenage health problems: Allies or adversaries? Presented at Family Impact Seminar, Washington, D.C., September 21, 1990.
10. Patterson GR, DeBaryshe BD, Ramsey E: A developmental perspective on antisocial behavior. Am Psychol 44:329, 1989.
11. Pelham WE, Carlson CL, Sams SE, et al: Separate and combined effects of methylphenidate and behavior modification on boys with attention deficit-hyperactivity disorder in the classroom. J Consult Clin Psychol 61:506, 1993.
12. Wills T: Help-seeking as a coping mechanism. In Snyder CR, Ford CE (eds): Coping with Negative Life Events. New York, Plenum Press, 1987.
13. York P, York D, Wachtel T: Toughlove. New York, Bantam Press, 1982.
14. York P, York D, Wachtel T: Toughlove Solutions. New York, Doubleday & Co., 1984.

The Medical Clinician's Roles in Preventing Adolescent Involvement in Violence

TRINA MENDEN ANGLIN, M.D., Ph.D.

Office of Adolescent Health
Maternal and Child Health Bureau
Health Resources and Services Administration
U.S. Public Health Service
Department of Health and Human Services
Rockville, Maryland

Reprint requests to:
Trina Menden Anglin, M.D., Ph.D.
Maternal and Child Health Bureau
Parklawn Building, Room 18A-39
5600 Fishers Lane
Rockville, MD 20857

EPIDEMIOLOGIC BACKGROUND

Many adolescents are exposed to interpersonal violence and participate in violent activities. They are at high risk for suffering and for causing serious psychological harm and irreparable physical harm, including death. Despite a decade of rising public concern and the development of prevention programming, adolescent violence and homicide rates remain very high, especially in impoverished communities. The most recently available statistics, however, suggest a possible encouraging downward trend.

Homicide

In general, homicide rates have been increasing among 15- to 19-year-olds since 1966, when the rate was measured at 5.1 per 100,000 population.[30] Rates have been at least 10.0 for this age group since 1986, when they started to climb sharply. Prevalence may have peaked in 1993, when the rate for males was 34.8 and the rate for females was 5.9 (total rate was 20.7 for this age group). Trend statistics are available for the age group 15–24 years, which combine rates for adolescents and young adults. Young adults (20–24 years) have an even higher homicide rate than adolescents (15–19 years). Annual rates per 100,000 15- to 24-year-olds for the 7-year period 1989–1995 were 16.9 in 1989, 19.9 in 1990, 22.4 in 1991, 22.2 in 1992, 23.4 in 1993, 19.8 in 1994, and 19.0 in 1995. These rates demonstrated a peak in 1993 and, most recently, a consistent 2-year decrease, which represents an 18.8% reduction between 1993 and 1995.[30]

Rates for male adolescents are about six times higher than those for female adolescents, and rates for nonwhite male teenagers (15–19 years old) are about 7.5 times greater than those for white male adolescents. Firearms remain the weapon of choice for homicide; in 1992, 87% of homicides among adolescents 15–19 years old were caused by firearms.[30]

The homicide rate is much lower for the younger adolescent age group. It was only 2.4 per 100,000 10- to 14-year-olds in 1992 (3.2 for young male and 1.6 for young female adolescents), 2.5 in 1993, and 1.7 per 100,000 in 1994.[30]

Fighting and Weapon Carrying

Additional evidence for progress in curtailing youthful violence comes from the Youth Risk Behavior Surveillance System, which is based on a national, representative sample of students in grades 9–12 who provide self-report information through classroom surveys.[15] It found significant decreases in the incidence of physical fighting between 1993 and 1995 among all students (incidence of 137 per 100 students per 12 months in 1993, which dropped to 128 in 1995). Similarly, weapon carrying by youth decreased significantly to an incidence of 81 per month per 100 students ages 14–17 since its 1991 baseline measurement of 107.[15]

Despite the encouraging decrease in incidence, significant proportions of adolescents continue to engage in behaviors that contribute to intentional injuries. The following information is summarized from the 1995 Youth Risk Behavior Survey.[15] Overall, 20% of students (31% of male, 8% of female) had carried a weapon such as a gun, knife, or club at least once during the 30 days preceding the survey. As students progressed from grade 9 to 12, they were less likely to carry weapons (23% of 9th graders and 16% of 12th graders). Almost 8% of all students had carried a gun, which included 12% of male and 2.5% of female students. Of all male students, 10% of white, 19% of black, and 17% of Hispanic students had carried a gun at least once in the 30 days preceding the survey.[15]

Large proportions of students reported being in a physical fight during the preceding year: 39% of all students, 46% of male students, and 31% of female students. Fighting was more common among 9th graders (47%) than among 12th grade students (31%). About 4% of students reported needing to receive medical treatment for injuries sustained during a physical fight, including 6% of male students and 2.5% of female students.[15]

Violence at School

Violence and violence-predisposing behaviors related to school were reported by large proportions of adolescents.[15] Almost 10% of students, including 14% of males and 5% of females, carried a weapon to school at least once during the 30 days preceding the survey. Students in the younger grades (11% of 9th graders) were more likely to carry weapons than students in more advanced grades (8% of 12th graders). Hispanics (14%) were more likely than white (9%) or black (10%) students to have carried a weapon on school property.[15] Almost 16% of students (21% of males and 10% of females) had been in a physical fight on school property during the preceding year. Such fighting involved more students in younger grade levels (22% of 9th graders) than advanced students (11% of 12th graders). Self-reported fighting was more common among Hispanic (21%) and black (20%) than white (13%) students.[15]

Students also reported significant rates of victimization related to school.[15] More than 8% of students (11% of males and 6% of females) had been threatened or injured with a weapon on school property during the preceding year. This was more common for students in younger grades (10% of 9th graders) than advanced grades (7% of 12th graders), and for Hispanic (12%) and black (11%) students than for white (7%) students. More than one-third (35%) of students reported that they had property stolen or deliberately damaged on school grounds during the preceding year. Male students

(41%) were more likely than female students (28%) to report property loss.[15] This type of victimization may precipitate physical retaliation.

The net effect of such violence was that more than 4% of students reported feeling too unsafe to attend school at least once during the 30 days preceding the survey. There were no gender differences. Close to 6% of 9th graders but only 3% of 12th graders reported such fear. About 8% of black and Hispanic students but only 3% of white students reported being too frightened to attend school.[15]

Victimization Rates

In the United States, adolescents have the highest victimization rates for crimes of violence (sexual assault, robbery, physical assault) of any age group. In 1994, 115 per 1000 12- to 15-year-olds and 122 per 1000 6- to 19-year olds were victimized by crimes of violence.[30] Adolescents also represent a significant proportion of child abuse and neglect cases. In 1994, 10- to 13-year-olds represented about 19% and 14- to 17-year olds composed almost 15% of all substantiated and indicated cases.[30]

Criminal Offenses

Adolescents represent the age group most likely to engage in criminal activities. In 1994, juvenile cases, which involve children younger than 18, composed about 22% of the total crime index, 14% of all violent crime, and 25% of all property crime.[16,30] This age group represented 31% of arrests for serious crimes and 24% of arrests for weapons charges. In 1993, the delinquency case rate disposed by the juvenile court system was 54.6 per 1000 youth. The age at referral to court was divided fairly evenly across each adolescent year, ages 13–17, with a range of 17–22% by each year of age. Based on the findings of a longitudinal study of national probability sample of youth, the National Youth Survey, whose subjects were at least 27 years old at the most recent wave of data collection, 17 years represents the peak age of committing serious offenses. At that age, about 25% of white and 36% of black males self-reported at least one serious violent offense irrespective of whether they had been arrested.[8] By official statistics, however, the age at which arrest rates peak for violent crime is about 18 years.[30]

Juvenile (ages 10–17) arrests for violent offenses and for weapon violations have increased significantly since the late 1980s. In particular, 1989 and 1992 witnessed major increases in juvenile arrests for several categories of offense. A reverse trend may be starting. In 1994, for the first time in several years, fewer juveniles were arrested for murder, forcible rape, and weapons violations. However, the total number of juvenile arrests for violent crime and for robbery and aggravated assault continued to increase.[16,30]

PREVENTION OF ADOLESCENT INVOLVEMENT IN VIOLENCE

It is clear from these statistics that all clinicians who provide care to adolescents will encounter patients who engage in behaviors that predispose to violence or who are victimized by violence. Given the magnitude of the societal problem of violence and its prominence as a public health issue, clinicians have a fiduciary obligation to prevent the morbidity and mortality associated with it. This chapter discusses how clinicians can become involved in the primary, secondary, and even tertiary prevention of violence and intervene with adolescents who have been victimized by violence. It also introduces preliminary information about the effectiveness of institutional and community-based efforts to treat adolescents involved in violence.

Clinicians' prevention activities can take place at two levels: individual clinical interactions with adolescents and their families and at the large group, or community, level. Two types of activities are important at the clinical level. Clinicians can identify three groups of teenagers who have been involved with violence: teenagers who are at risk for becoming involved in aggressive behaviors, teenagers who are already involved in seriously aggressive behaviors, and teenagers who have been victimized and may be suffering significant mental health sequelae. The clinician may be able to provide intervention for each category of teenager. The clinician can also become a powerful voice advocating for community investment in its youth.

IDENTIFICATION OF ADOLESCENTS INVOLVED WITH VIOLENCE

Clinicians may encounter and identify adolescents involved with violence in all usual sites of practice: offices, community health centers and hospital ambulatory care centers, emergency departments, and inpatient units, including intensive care and general inpatient services. Each major practice site, including outpatient, emergency department, and inpatient, should have protocols for routine use that aid in identifying, evaluating, and providing helpful interventions for adolescents at risk for future engagement in or victimization by violence.

Table 1 summarizes the content areas that should be addressed during the assessment of an adolescent's exposure to violence. This table includes questions about

TABLE 1. Clinical Screening of Adolescents for Exposure to Violence

Topic areas
- Beliefs and self-perceptions regarding aggression
- Direct victimization
- Witnessing and observing violence
- Aggression and perpetration of violence
- Chronology of exposure
- Sites of exposure (at home, at school, in the community)

Content areas
- Beliefs about aggression (legitimacy, whether it enhances social standing or image, attributions of hostile intent to others, victims do not suffer and deserve their victimization)
- Self-perceptions (impulsivity, anger, thrill-seeking, power)
- Peer relationships (cruel teasing or bullying, fighting and circumstances of fighting, observing fights as a bystander)
- Bias-motivated aggression as victim and as perpetrator (race/ethnicity, religion, sexual orientation)
- Threats of physical violence (threatening someone, being threatened)
- Chasing (chasing someone, being chased)
- Physical assaults (punching/hitting/kicking, being punched/hit/kicked; jumping/mugging/assaulting, being jumped/mugged/assaulted; robbing, being robbed)
- Weapon carrying (gun/knife/club or other, where carried, where/how obtained, techniques of storage, parental knowledge, reasons carried)
- Weapon use (shooting at someone and consequences, being shot at or shot, being caught in gunfire; attacking someone with a knife or club and consequences, being attacked by a knife or club)
- Within home (style of discipline, sense of safety and security within family, sense of nurturance and affection from parents, abuse/beating by parents, hitting parents/siblings, being hit by siblings, violence between/among home's adults, parents' beliefs about peer fighting)
- Gender role violence (between romantic partners, sexual harassment, fighting over a potential romantic partner)
- Sexual abuse or assault as a child or more recently (as victim, as perpetrator, including date rape)
- Physical injuries from fighting (what caused, what received)
- Finding a dead body or seriously injured person
- Physical safety (at and traveling to/from school, in the community, at work)
- Personal losses through violence (family members, friends, classmates, neighbors)
  - Emotional responses
  - Need to retaliate
  - Effects on other family members and friends

perpetration, witnessing, and victimization. The clinician will need to ask adolescent patients direct questions. Patients will not always volunteer this information but will usually answer honestly if asked. The clinician should consider an overlap of victimization and perpetration, especially if the teenager has witnessed considerable violence; carries a weapon, especially a gun; feels a need to retaliate or is chronically angry; or has had trouble with the police or the law.

Adolescents exposed to violence may develop mental health symptoms (Table 2).[11,23] They can present for clinical care in a variety of ways, but the cause of their symptoms is frequently hidden. Some adolescents present for treatment of physical injuries. This type of encounter provides an excellent opportunity for a more complete evaluation and initiation of intervention. An astute clinician can note incidental findings associated with trauma (e.g., bruising and scars) on physical examination during any type of visit; discussing the cause of an injury may offer an opportunity for intervention.

Teenagers seeking clinical preventive services and reproductive health care should be asked about possible exposure to violence as a routine part of the psychosocial profile. Elucidation of mental health concerns also may lead to a history of exposure to violence. Female teenagers may share information about their boyfriend's gunshot wound or homicide; the clinician may note ecchymoses from a romantic partner's physical assault.

Although the focus of this chapter is on adolescents involved in recent violence, many problem behaviors exhibited by adolescents may be associated with earlier and perhaps chronic exposure to violence, which may have occurred in the home. Examples of problem behaviors that have been empirically linked to child maltreatment include academic difficulty and school failure, substance abuse, having multiple sexual partners, running away, engaging in reckless and dangerous activities, suicide attempts and self-mutilation, a pugnacious and alienated attitude, delinquency, fighting, assaultive behavior, and other serious violent offenses.[5, 31]

Identification of Adolescents Exposed to Violence

About 25% of adolescents report being victimized by interpersonal violence,[10] and an unknown, but larger proportion have witnessed significant violence, which is called

TABLE 2. Mental Health Symptoms and Behaviors Associated with Adolescents' Exposure to Violence

- Disordered sleep (trouble initiating or maintaining sleep, hypersomnia, nightmares)
- Level of worrying
- Ability to concentrate and remember school lessons
- Thoughts that intrude or recur repeatedly
- Trying not to think or feel
- Feelings of being unreal or outside the real world looking in, being outside the body, being someone else, or that things or events don't seem real
- School attendance
- Changes in social activities
- Activities for fun
- Sadness, unhappiness, loneliness
- Significant increases or decreases in appetite
- Self-blame, guilt for unfortunate or bad events
- Feelings of safety/vulnerability
- Hope/despair
- Sense of future
- Suicidal ideation, plans, attempts
- Self-perceived irritability, anger levels, ability to control anger
- Substance use and perceived benefits of use

secondary victimization. Knowing someone who was seriously injured or murdered is also considered a form of secondary victimization.

Victimization by Hate-motivated Aggression

Certain groups of adolescents may be at especially high risk for victimization by violence. These youth may be targets of hate or bias-motivated bullying and crimes because of their race, ethnicity, religion, or sexual orientation. Adolescents victimized by hate-motivated aggression may not spontaneously report it because of stigma (e.g., homosexuality) or fear (e.g., of deportation if an illegal immigrant). Adolescents who belong to racial, ethnic, or religious groups that have densely populated a geographic area but do not compose the majority population may be at particular risk, both for being victimized by hate-motivated aggression (perhaps because they pose a threat to economic opportunities for the established population) and reciprocally for behaving aggressively, perhaps in retaliation, toward other groups.[17]

Mental Health Problems Associated with Exposure to Violence

Clinicians need to consider the possibility that exposure to violence caused a patient's mental health symptoms; conversely, they need to assess the mental health status of a patient who has been victimized by violence. There are several mental health problems associated with adolescents' exposure to violence.[23] These symptoms of psychological distress are outlined in Table 2 and may indicate anxiety, depression, existential despair, anger, or fear. Many of these problems can co-exist, especially anxiety and fear, anxiety and depression, and depression and anger.

ANXIETY

Anxiety frequently manifests as symptoms of physiologic arousal, which may include cardiac, respiratory, neurologic, and gastrointestinal symptoms. It may present as recurrent somatic symptoms or as panic attacks. It may take the form of a generalized anxiety that the patient has difficulty controlling or as separation anxiety.[2] Anxiety is frequently denied by symptomatic adolescent patients.

Posttraumatic stress disorder (PTSD) is an extreme form of anxiety disorder. It develops after a direct experience with or witnessing an intensely traumatic, surprising event that involved actual or threatened death or severe injury and that generated intense fear, helplessness, or horror. It causes significant distress and impairs social and academic functioning. (Acute stress disorder has a similar constellation of symptoms, but its time course is limited to 4 weeks). Stress disorders represented the most common mental health diagnosis in a set of urban high school-based student health centers.[3a] Three major symptoms are necessary for the diagnosis: persistent reexperiencing the event as intrusive thoughts or through dreams; persistent avoidance of associated stimuli and numbing of general responsiveness (e.g., active refusal to attend school, selective loss of memory about the event, feelings of detachment from others and decreased interest in activities, and inability to feel expressive emotion); and persistent symptoms of increased arousal such as hypervigilence, irritability, difficulty concentrating, and disturbed sleep.[1,2] More than 25% of children and adolescents who had been victims of or who had witnessed violence were found to have symptoms of PTSD.[11]

DEPRESSION

Depression is caused by recurrent losses and is reported more commonly by female than male adolescents. Its symptoms are well known and include a sad mood, decreased interest or pleasure in activities, significant changes in weight and in appetite, disturbed sleep (hypersomnia or insomnia), observable psychomotor agitation or retardation, fatigue or loss of energy, feelings of worthlessness or excessive guilt, and a diminished ability to concentrate and to make decisions. In addition, depressed adolescents may have thoughts of death or of suicide and may attempt suicide.[2] Adolescents exposed to violence may express existential despair and believe that their futures are foreshortened.[23]

ANGER

Anger is not a mental health diagnosis; it is a major feeling state that is commonly associated with exposure to violence and with depression. There is a strong empirical association between aggressive behavior and anger, and anger also has been linked to the use of weapons. Anger represents the mental health symptom most common in teenagers who have both perpetrated and been victimized by violence.[23] It is not uncommon for adolescents who are physically aggressive or who perpetrate violence to be at heightened risk for their own victimization.

FEAR

Although fear is not a formal mental health diagnosis, it can influence adolescents' behavior. Fear is a subjective feeling of impending harm or danger. Although it can be part of the symptoms of an anxiety disorder, fear is frequently based on realistic risks. It can cause constriction of adolescents' social experiences when it forces them to avoid dangerous places and situations. Adolescents exposed to violence may have a mixture of external bravado and internal fearfulness. The increased physiologic arousal induced by the anxiety of fear may create difficulty in modulating aggressive impulses, so that a belligerent responsiveness can become manifest.

Backgrounds of Adolescents Who Are Physically Aggressive

Physical aggression covers a range of behaviors. Many aggressive adolescents encountered by clinicians during routine office visits may get into fights or bully their peers but have not used weapons or become involved in behaviors that, if detected, would have resulted in their arrests. They may demonstrate some of the characteristics outlined below for adolescents who engage in seriously aggressive and violent behaviors. This latter group can be considered delinquent; this term is used by the justice system to describe antisocial behaviors of juveniles. Some may have an aggressive conduct disorder, which is a formal psychiatric diagnosis that implies a persistent and repetitive pattern of behavior that violates others' rights and societal rules.[2] There is a substantial overlap among adolescents who are aggressive, delinquent, and conduct-disordered. *Aggressiveness* is the most general term. However, when treatment options are outlined, the term *delinquent* is used because most programs have been evaluated on groups of adjudicated adolescents.

Aggressive adolescents commonly have the following attributes. First, their problems are frequently multiple; their aggressive behavior does not stand alone.[19,25,26] They are likely to perform poorly in school[12,13,28] and to abuse substances.[6,19,20] They may have additional comorbid psychiatric diagnoses such as attention deficit/hyperactivity disorder and depression.[6]

Adolescents at risk for seriously aggressive behavior frequently come from troubled families.[13,21,22,26,28] Many have been exposed to chronic intrafamilial violence and have received harsh and inconsistent discipline. At the same time, their families may not have provided sufficient structure and limit-setting; such permissiveness or lack of parental guidance prevents the development of self-control in children. This dual style of parenting has been found to contribute to the development of aggressiveness in children.

The families of these adolescents demonstrate low social cohesion, which results in little opportunity to receive nurturance or to forge a common familial identity. If their families have inadequate problem-solving skills, these adolescents may not have learned to address external demands (e.g., not enough money to support familial needs) effectively. Some family members may themselves model criminal behavior and have substance abuse problems.

These negative experiences at home create negative perceptions of the self and of other people. Adolescents with this background believe that people are generally hostile toward them, which creates a self-defensive leitmotif. The modeling of violence by family members, by neighborhood residents, and by peers helps to consolidate an aggressive style of behavior.[13,22] These youth have learned that aggression and violence are acceptable and normal and can be an effective and even a preferred method of dealing with conflict, even as exposure to both witnessed and experienced violence creates insecurity and psychological trauma.[26]

Aggressive adolescents frequently have impaired interpersonal relationships; they are rejected by most of their nonaggressive peers, and they refuse adult authority. Aggressive tendencies are reinforced when peers react strongly to bullying by these children; peers' hostility reifies aggressive children's and adolescents' beliefs. The developmental trajectory for males who eventually engage in violent behavior as older adolescents and young adults includes the earlier steps of bullying and other aggressive behaviors toward peers as children, followed by fighting and gang membership as younger adolescents. It is possible to predict by the primary grades which males will engage in violent behaviors as older adolescents and young adults.[13,14,18,21,22,28]

Aggressive adolescents' patterns of thought appear to be learned to such a degree that they become habitual and almost automatic. Their processes of thought appear to exclude effective social problem-solving skills. If a social problem occurs, the aggressive adolescent will define it as a hostile situation, attributing hostile intent to the other involved person, and will attempt to solve it using a hostile goal (e.g., "I will get you before you get me"). They are in a chronic state of self-defensiveness and readiness to self-protect through aggressive behavior. Aggressive adolescents do not have the cognitive flexibility to be able to generate alternative solutions to social problems or even to attempt to seek additional information about a problematic social situation that could help to modify their perspective about it. They hold several beliefs that are not shared by nonaggressive adolescents. They believe that aggression is a legitimate response to a social problem and that it enhances self-esteem and one's social image. Aggressive adolescents are not able to empathize with the suffering of victims and may even believe that victims deserve to be victimized. Stylistically, aggressive adolescents exhibit poor self-control. They are impulsive, especially when they are emotionally aroused, and are not able to think about situations in a reflective manner.[22,26,29] It is easy to see how a volatile situation may quickly provoke an aggressive response. In contrast to assumption, however, hopelessness has not been found to be associated with aggressive behavior.[14]

Many more adolescents observe aggressive encounters as bystanders than become directly involved. It is now known, however, that bystanders play important roles in the development and escalation of fights. Their presence frequently encourages the participants, and they may add vocal support to the fighters or even become physically involved in the fight. Bystanders to fights frequently share the same beliefs regarding violence and aggression that are outlined above and are likely to be socially rejected by their peers. Their thought patterns are not very different from those in adolescents who become directly engaged in aggression.[24]

In contrast, adolescents who are not aggressive and who refuse to watch a fight or help to prevent it are usually strongly accepted by their peers. They are able to generate prosocial solutions to interpersonal problems, to appreciate the perspectives of other parties in a dispute, to gather information about a problem as a step toward solving it, to behave reflectively rather than impulsively, and to behave assertively in a way that promotes the dignity of each party.[24] It is these skills that violence prevention and treatment programs try to teach children and adolescents.

PROVIDING CLINICAL INTERVENTIONS

Helping Adolescent Victims

To help adolescent victims who have been victimized by violence, the clinician needs to consider a variety of factors:

- Ask patients about issues of violence. Use an honest and straightforward approach; this style helps the adolescent to build trust in the clinician.
- Help the adolescent to appreciate that having emotional responses to violence is understandable and universal.
- Interpret symptoms of physiologic arousal as the body's normal response to a stressful and upsetting situation.
- Prepare the adolescent for an expected emotional course; psychological responses to violence take time to resolve.
- Help the adolescent and family to solve problems regarding physical safety. How can the adolescent get to and from school and around the neighborhood?
- Determine the need for referral for formal mental health evaluation and treatment. Consider the symptoms' intensity, frequency, duration, and pervasiveness. How much do symptoms interfere with functioning? What degree of distress and suffering are they causing? Early mental health intervention may be able to prevent or ameliorate maladaptive coping.
- Consider the availability of wise, nurturing familial support. A family may not be available because of its members' own traumatization, depression, or substance use.

Clinicians need to become familiar with their communities' violence prevention and mental health resources. Ensuring that an individual mental health professional is skilled in working with adolescents and can recognize when psychopharmacotherapy is needed would be helpful. Today, many community mental health centers, prosocial organizations, and religious congregations offer teen support groups. Schools may offer counseling and other support services. Unjudicated adolescents at risk for perpetration who present as victims of violence may do well in certain court diversion programs. Juvenile gang unit officers may be particularly knowledgeable about a community's resources for teenagers.

The clinician should maintain contact with the adolescent and family, continue to act in a supportive role, and ensure successful completion of and continued engagement with a mental health professional. If an adolescent or family is reluctant to accept referral for mental health care, the clinician should establish the parameters that dictate its necessity. For example, if an adolescent's symptoms of anxiety or depression continue to interfere with daily school attendance and the ability to actively participate in extracurricular activities despite a supportive parental presence, mental health intervention is mandatory.

Preventing Adolescent Involvement in Violence

To provide the most meaningful prevention and intervention at the clinical and community advocacy levels, the clinician should know which types of approaches may be helpful, ineffective, or even counterproductive. Although multiple approaches and programs have been developed, formal evaluation efforts have been limited, especially for primary and secondary prevention programs.

PRIMARY VIOLENCE PREVENTION PROGRAMS

The goal of primary prevention programs is to prevent aggressive and violent behaviors.[13,22,29,32] They are usually conducted for groups, such as classrooms of students or youth members of recreational clubs. They promote prosocial behavior and competency through psychoeducational programs and can modify group norms regarding such issues as the value of fighting and can increase group skills in avoiding physical confrontation among peers. However, their strategies, although not well studied, may be more effective for children and early adolescents. As described above, because fighting and weapon carrying are significantly more common among younger than older school-attending adolescents, it is appropriate to aim these efforts at younger students. There are two possible reasons for this observation. The first is that adolescents stop fighting as they mature. The second is that adolescents who continue these activities may drop out of school and, therefore, would not be included in the 12th grade sample.

Although different curricula have been developed, they are often based on a problem-solving model that is governed by the principles that adolescents have the internal resources to solve interpersonal problems, that mutual respect should guide everyone's interactions, that each party has a responsibility to listen, and that each party has a right to be heard.[9] The curricula provide students with the opportunity to practice considering optimal responses to interpersonal situations by using different sources of information, looking at possible consequences, making the decision to act, and evaluating the outcome of the situation based on their personal values. These programs have been covered in detail by Wilson-Brewer[32] and are not discussed further in this chapter except as they can be adapted for use by health care clinicians.

The six steps of the sample curriculum[9] outlined in Table 3 form the acronym SCIDDLE; they can be adapted for use in an office-based practice and can be used to help consolidate learning from a school-based curriculum or to help adolescents who get into fights impulsively. (In this case, this strategy would be considered secondary violence prevention.) A specific scenario that a clinician can use to frame the SCIDDLE steps with adolescent patients who get into fights is the example of being bumped in the hallway by another teenager. Although such incidents are frequently nonintentional and would be interpreted by most adolescents as being inconsequential and without specific meaning, aggressive adolescents may assume that being bumped represents a hostile intent. They are likely to quickly—almost reflexively—display retaliatory aggression and feel justified in doing so. The clinician's tasks are to help the patient recognize that being bumped may be beyond volitional control and that becoming angry and retaliating is not a justifiable or an appropriate response and, also, to help the patient learn how to gather additional information before deciding to act.

SECONDARY VIOLENCE PREVENTION PROGRAMS

Secondary violence prevention programs attempt to mitigate the further development of serious aggressive behaviors in individuals with early manifestations.[13,29] They address risk factors and markers and should be tailored to individuals' specific needs.[27] Successful programs attempt to address the constellation of markers associated with adolescents involved in aggressive behaviors.[13] A multimodal approach is usually necessary.[27] These factors include low self-control and familial dysfunction that includes aversive styles of parenting, poor school performance, inability to get along with mainstream

TABLE 3. Practical Suggestions for Clinicians

FOR SITE OF CARE

For clinical practice setting

Ensure that the clinical preventive services protocol includes

- A strategy to screen adolescents for psychosocial functioning, including school performance, familial dynamics, and substance use and abuse
- Questions about involvement in violence as a victim and as a perpetrator
- Questions about firearms in the home and familial beliefs about firearms
- A mechanism for referring appropriate patients and families for more complete evaluation and tailored intervention services

During patient encounters

As part of anticipatory guidance, discuss with families and adolescents

- Consistent limit-setting and application of family rules, supervision, discipline style, and behavior management
- Having gun-free homes
- Becoming active bystanders who do not support fights and who try to deescalate tense interpersonal situations
- Having the moral courage to speak out on behalf of peers who are being bullied or scapegoated
- Importance of nonviolent romantic relationships and how to recognize abuse within dating relationships

For adolescents at risk for victimization on basis of race/ethnicity, religion, sexual orientation

- Become active in school's peer mediation program; learn how to negotiate and to mediate conflicts
- Join mainstream school activities and the student government
- Enroll in a self-defense course to help build self-confidence

For adolescents who initiate fights or who get into frequent fights

Additional interactive evaluation questions that can lead to intervention

- Determine what benefits fighting is perceived as having
- Determine whether the adolescent ever feels remorse for fighting
- Determine the adolescent's self-image and perceptions of image that others have of him/her (Is renown for fighting the only way the adolescent feels he/she can gain peer respect?)
- Determine adolescent's awareness of violence prevention efforts around the country and in own community. What are these programs trying to teach, and how might the adolescent apply their principles?
- Consider whether adolescent may have attention deficit/hyperactivity disorder that had not been previously identified.
- Assess adolescent for use of tobacco, alcohol, and other drugs

Intervention strategies

- Work with patient, parents, and school regarding behavioral contracting for fighting behavior and school performance
- Work with adolescent using a problem-solving approach (acronym SCIDDLE)[9]
    - **S**top and assess a possibly provocative situation. Do not react impulsively.
    - **C**alm down. Assess your emotional state. Do not react based on intense emotions.
    - **I**dentify the problem and how you feel about it.
    - **D**ecide, or determine, your options, and consider the consequences of each. There are four prosocial options open for adolescents to use, which form the acronym RAID: **r**esolve, **a**void, **i**gnore, and **d**iffuse (e.g., use gentle humor).
    - **D**o it. Take action.
    - **L**ook back and **E**valuate. How well did your approach work? Was it congruent with your values, how you want to see yourself, and how you want others to see you?
- Advance adolescent's sociomoral reasoning
- Help the adolescent to develop the belief that it is wrong to harm others, and reinforce that this belief is important to hold
- Help the adolescent to become empathetic to victims and to appreciate the universality of pain
- Help the adolescent to see interpersonal problems from the perspective of each party and to work out a solution that is fair to each

For hospital

- Ensure that the emergency department uses a protocol to determine the contextual causes of all adolescent injuries and provides appropriate intervention services for youth (and for their families and friends) involved in violence as either perpetrators or victims
- Ensure that inpatient units use a protocol for evaluating all admitted adolescents (including adolescents admitted with trauma, medical, and psychiatric problems) for involvement in violence and provide appropriate intervention services

Continued on next page.

TABLE 3. Practical Suggestions for Clinicians *(Continued)*

FOR COMMUNITY
• Learn what violence prevention efforts exist. Determine whether the models on which they are based have been evaluated for efficacy, and whether they have been found to be effective. Schools, juvenile court, and the police frequently have developed violence prevention programs.
• Promote parenting support and guidance programs and opportunities for positive familial interaction
• Support programs that provide children and adolescents with opportunities for development of life and social skills, humanitarianism, and citizenship skills
• Ensure that the school district has a policy about bullying and that this problem is taken seriously by school personnel, so that schoolwide prevention programming is in place and that constructive intervention is routinely available for bullies and victims

peers, and association with other aggressive teens.[13] In addition, they attempt to modify the environment to make aggressive behavior less normative and tolerable (e.g, a school's anti-bullying campaign). They also address such coexisting problems as substance abuse. They may work to promote constructive leadership opportunities for youth at risk.

Referral of families to programs that work on parenting and internal communication skills has been successful for younger and middle adolescents.[7,13,28] (If they are continued long-term, these programs may be even more successful for children identified as being aggressive during early elementary school and therefore at risk for delinquency and conduct disorder as they become older.[22,28]) These programs help parents to apply principles of social learning to the upbringing and discipline of their children and to increase their supervision of their children's activities.[7,13] Clinicians can locate such programs through school guidance counselors, juvenile court, the community's department of human services, and local university departments of psychology.

Clinicians also can help their adolescent patients to succeed at school. Most directly, the clinician can contact the student's guidance counselor to advocate for constructive attention; specifically, the student could be included in specialized programming or considered for alternative placement.[12] The clinician may be able to motivate the parents to become invested in their adolescent's education and behavior while at school. A four-way contract among school, clinician, parents, and adolescent may be helpful in improving academic interest and behavior. Comprehensive familial programs for adolescents at risk for delinquency may also include a component for improving school performance.[4,13,27]

It may be challenging to engage parents successfully in secondary prevention efforts.[13] A genetic influence on antisocial behavior is probable, and it is intertwined with learned parenting style.[6] In addition, most of these adolescents' parents probably did not themselves enjoy a successful academic experience, and they may feel alienated from schools.

Secondary prevention programs may use the same approach described above and outlined in Table 3 for building social competence in difficult interpersonal situations. However, the work may be more intensive.

Secondary prevention programs also attempt to limit their adolescent clients' associations with delinquent peers. It is difficult to achieve this goal for teenagers, who have already chosen their peer groups.[13] Strategies include helping parents to supervise their children's activities more closely and encouraging adolescents to develop interests and talents in such constructive activities as art, music, dance, photography, and mechanics. Mentorship programs, although not well evaluated, may be a useful strategy for this objective. It may be important to limit social contact among aggressive or delinquent adolescents even in the context of treatment programs. At least two evaluations of experimental programs found that activities for groups of delinquent youth, no matter how constructive their intent, had the inadvertent consequence of increasing antisocial behavior or substance use.[7,18]

Substance abuse is common among aggressive adolescents[6,20] and represents a functional part of the definition of conduct disorder.[2] It is likely that many adolescents referred for substance abuse treatment actually have a conduct disorder that is not recognized by the treatment program.[6] As part of secondary prevention efforts, the clinician needs to address substance use problems.

TERTIARY VIOLENCE PREVENTION PROGRAMS

Tertiary-level programs provide intervention and treatment for the most seriously troubled adolescents as part of correctional and psychiatric programs. The goal is to prevent recidivism.[13] These efforts are the best evaluated types of programs.[29] Recent meta-analyses have demonstrated that compared to correctional institutions, community-based programs (e.g., day treatment programs, group homes, intensive at-home probation) with strong designs and competent, consistent, long-term application can positively influence recidivism rates.[3,13] However, many community treatment programs are not as strong as they could be and can actually allow increased rates of reoffending because they are not supervised as closely as are traditional institutions of correction.[13]

When treatment modalities are compared, those with vaguely formulated goals, such as traditional psychotherapy and casework, have not by themselves been found to be effective in preventing recidivism.[13,27,29] However, they may be helpful adjuncts[27,29] (e.g., psychotherapeutic approaches for depression). Cognitive-behavioral approaches aimed at adolescents and their families, as outlined above, have generally been found to have some short-term success.[13,27,29] However, positive effects may diminish when youth return home; long-term treatment appears essential for maintaining progress. The programs that have long-term success are multimodal and provide interventions that focus on the adolescent, family, school, neighborhood, and peer group.[4,27]

The office-based clinician can become part of the community-based adjudicated adolescent's treatment team by providing continuity of care, communicating clearly in writing to the program, and contacting the adolescent's case manager with any concerns. The clinician can be helpful by determining the adolescent's self-perception of progress and adaptation to the program. The clinician can check to ensure that familial and scholastic components of the patient's treatment program are taking place, that issues of substance abuse are being addressed, and that other comorbid conditions, such as attention deficit/hyperactivity disorder, have been identified.

CONCLUSION

Concern about high levels of adolescent involvement in violence has prompted the development of prevention programs. Given the high prevalence of violence, clinicians need to learn how to identify adolescent victims, recognize mental health sequelae, and to provide intervention. In working with adolescents who are physically aggressive and at risk for more serious involvement in violence, clinicians can adapt the principles of cognitively-based prevention programs for office use. Clinicians can help by referring these patients to community-based secondary prevention programs and advocating for comprehensive, effective treatment modalities. They need to ensure that major comorbid conditions associated with aggressive behavior, including substance abuse and attention deficit/hyperactivity disorder, are identified and treated.

Clinicians should also ensure that policies are in place at their sites of practice and hospitals that can enhance the identification and treatment of adolescents involved in violence. Finally, they can advocate with their school districts and communities to ensure that constructive policies and programs exist that address the primary, secondary, and tertiary prevention of violence among youth.

References

1. Amaya-Jackson L, March JS: Post-traumatic stress disorder in adolescents: Risk factors, diagnosis, and intervention. Adolesc Med State Art Rev 6:251–269, 1995.
2. American Psychiatric Association: Diagnostic and Statistical Manual of Mental Disorders, 4th ed. Washington, DC, American Psychiatric Association, 1994.
3. Andrews DA, Zinger I, Hoge RD, et al: Does correctional treatment work? A clinically relevant and psychologically informed meta-analysis. Criminology 28:369–404, 1990.

3a. Anglin TM, Naylor KE, Kaplan DW: Comprehensive school-based health care: High school students' utilization of medical, mental health, and substance abuse services. Pediatrics 97:318–330, 1996.

4. Borduin CM, Cone LT, Mann BJ, et al: Multisystemic treatment of serious juvenile offenders: Long-term prevention of criminality and violence. J Consult Clin Psychol 63:569–578, 1995.
5. Council on Scientific Affairs, American Medical Association: Adolescents as victims of family violence. JAMA 270:1850–1856, 1993.
6. Crowley TJ, Riggs PD: Adolescent substance use disorder with conduct disorder and comorbid conditions. In Rahdert E, Czechowicz C (eds): Adolescent Drug Abuse: Clinical Assessment and Therapeutic Interventions. Rockville, MD, National Institute on Drug Abuse, 1995, pp 49–111.
7. Dishion TJ, Andrews DW: Preventing escalation in problem behaviors with high-risk young adolescents: Immediate and 1-year outcomes. J Consult Clin Psychol 63:538–548, 1995.
8. Elliott DS: Serious violent offenders: Onset, developmental course, and termination—the American Society of Criminology 1993 Presidential Address. Criminology 32:1–21, 1994.
9. Farrell AD, Meyer AL, Dahlberg LL: Richmond youth against violence: A school-based program for urban adolescents. Am J Prev Med 12(suppl 2):13–21, 1996.
10. Finkelhor D, Dzuiba-Leatherman J: Children as victims of violence: A national survey. Pediatrics 94:413–420, 1994.
11. Fitzpatrick KM, Boldizar JP: The prevalence and consequences of exposure to violence among African-American youth. J Am Acad Child Adolesc Psychiatry 32:419–423, 1993.
12. Goldstein AP, Harootunian B, Conoley JC: Student Aggression: Prevention, Management and Replacement Training. New York, The Guilford Press, 1994.
13. Gottfredson DC, Sealock MD, Koper CS: Delinquency. In DiClemente RJ, Hansen WB, Ponton LE (eds): Handbook of Adolescent Health Risk Behavior. New York, Plenum Press, 1996, pp 259–288.
14. Guerra NG, Tolan PH, Huesmann LR, et al: Stressful events and individual beliefs as correlates of economic disadvantage and aggression among urban children. J Consult Clin Psychol 63:518–528, 1995.
15. Kann L, Warren CW, Harris WA, et al: Youth risk behavior surveillance—United States, 1995. MMWR 45(SS-4):3,6–8,32–40, 1996.
16. Maguire K, Pastore AL (eds): Bureau of Justice Statistics Sourcebook of Criminal Justice Statistics—1995. Washington, DC, U.S. Department of Justice, Bureau of Justice Statistics, 1996.
17. Maxwell C, Maxwell SR: Youth Participation in Hate-Motivated Crimes: Research and Policy Implications. Boulder, CO, Center for the Study and Prevention of Violence, Institute for Behavioral Sciences, University of Colorado, 1995.
18. McCord J, Tremblay RE (eds): Preventing Antisocial Behavior: Interventions from Birth through Adolescence. New York, The Guilford Press, 1992.
19. O'Donnell J, Hawkins JD, Abbott RD: Predicting serious delinquency and substance use among aggressive boys. J Consult Clin Psychol 63:529–537, 1995.
20. Osgood DW: Drugs, alcohol, and adolescent violence. Boulder, CO, Center for the Study and Prevention of Violence, Institute for Behavioral Sciences, University of Colorado, 1995.
21. Pepler DJ, Rubin KH (eds): The Development and Treatment of Childhood Aggression. Hillsdale, NJ, Lawrence Erlbaum Associates, 1991.
22. Rivara FP, Farrington DP: Prevention of violence. Role of the pediatrician. Arch Pediatr Adolesc Med 149:421–429, 1995.
23. Singer MI, Anglin TM, Song L, Lunghofer L: Adolescents' exposure to violence and associated symptoms of psychological trauma. JAMA 273:477–482, 1995.

24. Slaby RG, Stringham P: Prevention of peer and community violence: The pediatrician's role. Pediatrics 94(suppl 4):608–616, 1994.
25. Sosin DM, Koepsell TD, Rivara FP, Mercy JA: Fighting as a marker for multiple behaviors in adolescents. J Adolesc Health 16:209–215, 1995.
26. Staub E: Cultural-societal roots of violence. The examples of genocidal violence and of contemporary youth violence in the United States. Am Psychologist 51:117–132, 1996.
27. Tate DC, Reppucci ND, Mulvey EP: Violent juvenile delinquents. Treatment effectiveness and implications for future action. Am Psychologist 50:777–781, 1995.
28. Tolan PH, Guerra NG, Kendall PC: A developmental-ecological perspective on antisocial behavior in children and adolescents: Toward a unified risk and intervention framework. J Consult Clin Psychol 63:579–584, 1995.
29. Tolan P, Guerra N: What works in reducing adolescent violence: An empirical review of the field. Boulder, CO, Center for the Study and Prevention of Violence, Institute for Behavioral Sciences, University of Colorado, 1994.
30. U.S. Bureau of the Census: Statistical Abstract of the United States, 1996, 116th ed. Washington, DC, U.S. Government Printing Office, 1996.
31. Widom CS: Childhood victimization and adolescent problem behaviors. In Ketterlinus RD, Lamb ME (eds): Adolescent Problem Behaviors: Issues and Research. Hillsdale, NJ, Lawrence Erlbaum Associates, 1994, pp 127–164.
32. Wilson-Brewer R: Peer prevention programs in middle and high schools. Adolesc Med State Art Rev 6:233–250, 1995.

How Should Pediatricians Approach the Depressed Adolescent?

JEFF Q. BOSTIC, M.D., Ed.D.
TIMOTHY E. WILENS, M.D.

Department of Psychiatry
Harvard Medical School
and
Pediatric Psychopharmacology Clinic
Massachusetts General Hospital
Boston, Massachusetts

Reprint requests to:
Jeff Q. Bostic, M.D., Ed.D.
Massachusetts General Hospital
15 Parkman Street
WAC 725
Boston, MA 02114-3139

I was a seriously depressed kid. Every night at one point I'd go to bed bawling my head off. I used to try to make my head explode by holding my breath, thinking if I blew up my head, they'd be sorry . . . I wanted to die . . . I wanted to smash things.

—Kurt Cobain, Nirvana's lead singer, who committed suicide in 1994[32]

Confronted with despondent adolescents, pediatricians are increasingly required to distinguish youth pained by the developmental challenges of adolescence from youth suffering a mood disorder such as depression. Depression debilitates adolescents, impairing development in all arenas of life. Depressed adolescents describe falling self-esteem, conflicts with parents and peers, and problems with school behavior and achievement. Yet once these adolescents are properly identified and treated, such deficits diminish.[23] Pediatricians thus are expected to make accurate diagnoses and prescribe cost-efficient treatments, including when to treat and when to refer. These adolescents present substantial challenges to the pediatrician. This chapter reviews the most common dilemmas and treatment alternatives.

MOOD DISORDERS

Mood, the sustained feeling coloring a person's view of the world, greatly affects how one experiences events. Adolescents describe pervasive and persisting distressful moods such as severe sadness (the hallmark of major depressive disorder, or MDD); milder, but chronic sadness (dysthymia); and elevated, euphoric moods (mania or bipolar disorder).

TABLE 1. DSM–IV Criteria for Selected Mood Disorders

Major Depressive Episode
Five or more of the following symptoms have been present, by subjective report or observation by others, during the same 2-week period and represent a change from previous functioning; at least one of the symptoms is either (1) depressed mood or (2) loss of interest or pleasure. These symptoms should be present most of the day, nearly every day, cause clinically significant distress or functional impairment, and not be attributable to a general medical condition or effects of a substance.

(1) Depressed or irritable mood
(2) Markedly diminished interest or pleasure in almost all activities
(3) Significant weight loss or gain, or decrease or increase in appetite
(4) Insomnia or hypersomnia
(5) Psychomotor agitation or retardation
(6) Fatigue or loss of energy
(7) Feelings of worthlessness or excessive or inappropriate guilt
(8) Diminished ability to think or concentrate, or indecisiveness
(9) Recurrent thoughts of death (not fear of dying), recurrent suicidal ideation without a specific plan, or a suicide attempt or specific plan for committing suicide

Manic Episode
A distinct period of abnormally and persistently elevated, expansive, or irritable mood, lasting at least 1 week (or any duration if hospitalization is necessary). During this period, *three* or more of the following symptoms (four, if mood is only irritable) have been present to a significant degree. These symptoms should cause clinically significant distress or functional impairment, and not be attributable to a general medical condition or effects of a substance. If the mood disturbance does not cause marked impairment, necessitate hospitalization, or occur with psychotic features, then the mood disturbance is classified as a *hypomanic* episode.

(1) Inflated self-esteem
(2) Decreased need for sleep
(3) More talkative than usual or pressure to keep talking
(4) Flight of ideas or subjective experience that thoughts are racing
(5) Distractibility (i.e., attention too easily drawn to unimportant or irrelevant external stimuli)
(6) Increase in goal-directed activity or psychomotor agitation
(7) Excessive involvement in pleasurable activities that have high potential for painful consequences

Dysthymic Disorder
Depressed or irritable mood most of the day, for more days than not, as indicated by subjective account or observation by others for at least one year, and cause clinically significant distress or functional impairment. A major depressive or manic/hypomanic episode has not been present during this interval, the disturbance does not occur exclusively during the course of a psychotic disorder, the symptoms are not attributable to another medical condition or the effects of a substance, and the person has never been without the symptoms for more than 2 months at a time. Two or more of the following symptoms accompany the depressed mood:

(1) Poor appetite or overeating
(2) Insomnia or hypersomnia
(3) Low energy or fatigue
(4) Low self-esteem
(5) Poor concentration or indecisiveness
(6) Feelings of hopelessness

Mood disorders can be distinguished based on specific symptom constellations.[16] The diagnostic criteria for mood and other disorders can be found in the new pediatrician-friendly version of *The Diagnostic and Statistical Manual–IV*.[7] The current *DSM–IV* criteria for major depression, mania, and dysthymia are presented in Table 1.

Adolescent mood disorders are more common than previously presumed, and their prevalence appears to be increasing. MDD or dysthymia occurs in 5–10% of adolescents, and bipolar disorder affects 0.5–1%.[20] While boys outnumber girls with MDD prepubertally, by adolescence the distribution shifts to girls outnumbering boys 2:1.

IDENTIFICATION AND DIAGNOSIS OF MOOD DISORDERS

Clinical interviewing most effectively identifies adolescents with mood disorders. Beyond the symptoms listed in Table 1, adolescents frequently describe atypical depressive symptoms such as mood-reactivity (oversensitivity to mild environmental events), hyperphagia, hypersomnia, excessive fatiguability, and rejection-sensitivity (overreaction to perceived rejections).[14]

Most depressed adolescents also have comorbid psychiatric disorders, typically an anxiety disorder.[1] One-third of adolescents simultaneously have chronic milder dysthymia and episodes of severe major depression, which is called double depression. Substance abuse and conduct disorder may be present in depressed adolescents and may respond favorably to the treatment of the underlying mood disorder.[16]

The medical history may further help identify an adolescent with a mood disorder. Since many depressed adolescents are brought to the pediatrician because of excessive or recurrent somatic complaints, the pediatrician should consider possible mood disturbance when no cause of the symptoms is apparent. Conversely, hypothyroidism or hypocalcemia may manifest as depression, and hyperthyroidism or seizure disorders may resemble mania. Iatrogenic causes also warrant consideration. For example, some antihypertensives (e.g., clonidine, propanolol) or anticonvulsants (e.g., phenobarbital) may be depressogenic, and corticosteroids may cause conspicuous mood fluctuations.

Since mood disorders are highly familial, the pediatrician may benefit from eliciting family history. Because parents are sometimes reluctant to divulge to their children the mental health treatment of family members, this information may be better obtained when the adolescent is not present. Depressed adolescents are twice as likely to have a parent or sibling with depression or alcoholism.[29] Moreover, the younger a person manifests a mood disorder, the greater the likelihood that first-degree relatives also have a mood disorder.[33]

Evaluation of the impacts of the depression on the adolescent's functioning with peers, within the family, and at school may illuminate a mood disorder. Inability to maintain peer relationships, disinterest in activities previously enjoyed with peers, or withdrawal from friends may accompany depression. Withdrawal from family activities, missing meals, sleeping through family rituals, failing to complete chores, or unprovoked aggression often follow mood deterioration. Changes related to school, such as falling grades, increased behavioral problems or absences, incomplete homework, or withdrawal from school activities may signal a mood disturbance.

Although diagnoses of mood disorders rest on the clinical interview, other measures may augment the clinical history. Laboratory testing is obtained consonant with clinical suspicion. Blood chemistries are obtained when specific medical causes are suspected. Neuroendocrine challenge tests are currently used only in research domains. Neuroimaging is indicated when an abnormal neurologic or physical examination suggests focal lesions or, also, with the sudden onset of psychosis. Self-report measures, screening instruments, or rating scales (such as the Child Behavior Checklist and Child Depression Inventory) may identify additional mood disorder symptoms, elucidate comorbid disorders, and may be useful in monitoring treatment.

DURATION OF DEPRESSION

Adolescents usually recover from depressive episodes in 7–9 months. Of those entering treatment, more than 70% recover within a year. Unfortunately, mood disorders are frequently chronic and recurrent; almost three-fourths of depressed adolescents will have a subsequent depressive episode.[16] Many adolescents require chronic antidepressant treatment and require vigilant follow-up to minimize functional impairment from relapses or recurrent episodes.

Among the most disconcerting problems faced by pediatricians managing depressed adolescents is the possibility of the adolescent developing a more disabling bipolar disorder. "Switching" from depression to mania occurs in 20–33% of adolescents initially diagnosed with depression, usually within 6 months, and is not related to medication exposure.[12] These manic symptoms may emerge insidiously, often with irritability that progresses to erratic goal-directed but unproductive behavior, and culminating with decreasing sleep, severe outbursts, and inability to distinguish reality from fantasy. Predictors of manic switching include family history of bipolar disorder, prominent motoric changes, psychosis, and rapid onset of depressive symptoms.[5]

ASSESSING THE SUICIDAL ADOLESCENT

Suicidal thoughts and behavior are frequent among depressed adolescents. The Centers for Disease Control and Prevention estimates that 8% of high school students make serious suicide attempts each year. Although chronic depression and bipolar disorder are the most common diagnoses of those who attempt suicide,[20] one-third of those who complete suicide have been depressed less than 3 months when they committed suicide.[6]

Risk factors for suicidality include poor social adjustment, current mood disorder, substance abuse, impulsivity, psychological trauma, and delinquency. Relationship variables increasing suicide risk include recent rejections, humiliation, recent arguments, loss of a parent, and family discord.[22] Adolescents exposed to another's suicide have been inhibited from committing suicide themselves.[6] Neurobiologically, the most consistent findings in suicidal patients are low serotonin levels regardless of psychiatric diagnosis.[21] Despite concerns regarding overdose, antidepressants significantly decrease suicide risk.

Although unfounded, physicians often fear that questioning the adolescent about suicide may provoke suicidal thoughts or acts. Accordingly, clinicians should investigate and explore suicidality with the adolescent and, if denied but still suspected, with relatives, peers, and teachers. Asking about circumstances surrounding suicidal thoughts, previous suicidal experiences, reasons for suicide, and suicidal fantasies (e.g., what the adolescent imagines would happen if he attempted suicide or how others would react if he died) may reveal suicidal motivations that can be addressed effectively. The use of available interventions also can reduce suicidal behaviors. Specifically, suicidality decreases when a support network is cultivated that reduces stress, observes for signs of impending suicidal acts, and allows ventilation of distressing feelings.[22]

Access to means of suicide warrants assessment since most youth suicides occur with firearms[6] or household medications. Potentially lethal items should be removed from the household. If parents lack the capacity to ensure safety and remove means to suicide, hospitalization of the adolescent may be required.

PSYCHOTHERAPY

Psychotherapy may be preferred for some depressed adolescents. For example, studies in adults show that psychotherapy and pharmacotherapy yield similar results in mild to moderate depressions. Adolescents with identified stressors precipitating their mood changes and adolescents who are experiencing changes in family, friends, or schooling and are exhibiting persistent dysfunctional or self-destructive patterns may benefit from psychotherapy.

No controlled studies of psychotherapy using rigorous assessments or follow-up have been conducted with mood-disordered adolescents, but retrospective reviews showed benefit for intensive psychotherapy among youth.[9] More time-focused "manual" treatments such as cognitive-behavioral therapy (CBT) and interpersonal therapy (IPT) offer alternative treatments for depression. Although additional data are needed to clarify the specific benefits and applications of psychotherapy, it remains the standard of care in the treatment of depressed adolescents.

ANTIDEPRESSANTS

Response by Adolescents

To best understand pharmacotherapy in depressed adolescents, it is necessary to review the literature (Table 2). Open studies of antidepressants in adolescents showed response rates of approximately 75%,[4] but subsequent controlled studies generated less enthusiasm for antidepressant treatments of depressed adolescents.

Table 2 reveals that antidepressant efficacy is impeded by high placebo response rates. Studies of the tricyclic antidepressants (TCAs) amitriptyline, desipramine, and nortriptyline in adolescents showed that (1) the various TCAs had no significant advantage over placebo, (2) higher drug levels were associated with worsening of depression symptoms, and (3) larger studies were discontinued when few patients responded but none of the studies reported significant discontinuation because of side effects or EKG changes.

Two controlled trials of serotonin reuptake inhibitor (SRI) have been completed, yielding optimistic findings. Although Simeon et al. found a high placebo response, significant improvements in almost all depressive symptoms were greater on fluoxetine than placebo, and side effects were usually mild and transient.[27] A larger trial by Emslie et al. resulted in more robust support for fluoxetine in depressed adolescents.[8] Additional support is needed to corroborate these findings, and multisite adolescent depression trials with SRIs such as paroxetine and sertraline are in progress.

Prescription of Antidepressants

For adolescents diagnosed with MDD and experiencing substantial impairment, an antidepressant may be prescribed by the clinician (Table 3). Augmentation with psychotherapy or collaboration with mental health professionals is also recommended.

TABLE 2. Controlled Studies of Antidepressant Treatment of Adolescents

					Results	
Study	**N**	**Agent**	**Dose**	**Length (wk)**	**Active (%)**	**Placebo (%)**
Kramer and Feiguine, 1981[17]	20	Amitriptyline	200 mg/day	6	80	60
Geller et al., 1990[11]	35	Nortriptyline	80 ± 20 ng/ml	8	8	21
Koplewicz and Klein, 1990[15]	30	Desipramine	≤ 5 mg/kg/day	6	60	40
Simon et al., 1990[27]	40	Fluoxetine	60 mg/day	7	66	66
Kutcher et al., 1994[18]	60	Desipramine	200 mg/day	6	48	35
Kye et al, 1996[19]	31	Amitriptyline	5 mg/kg/day	8	75* 92†	30* 90†
Emslie et al, 1997[8]	96	Fluoxetine	20 mg/day	8	56	33

* Hamilton Depression Scale score < 6.
† Hamilton Depression Scale reduction > 50%.

TABLE 3. Antidepressants Used with Adolescents

Agent	Indications	Dosing: Initial (mg)	Dosing: Target (mg/kg/day)	Schedule
Serotonin reuptake inhibitors				
Fluoxetine	Major depression, dysthymia, obsessive-compulsive disorder, anorexia nervosa, bulimia, generalized anxiety	10–20 qam	0.25–0.70	qd–bid
Paroxetine		5–10 qam	0.25–0.70	qd–bid
Sertraline		25–50 qam	1.5–3	qd–bid
Fluvoxamine		25–50 qhs	1.5–4.5	bid
Atypical antidepressants				
Bupropion	Major depression, ADHD, bipolar depression	37.5 qam	3–6	tid (SR: qd–bid)
Venlafaxine	Major depression, ADHD	25 qam	2–3	bid–tid
Nefazodone	Major depression + anxiety	25–50 bid	4–8	bid
Trazodone	Sleep disorders	12.5–50 qhs	2–4	qhs–bid
Tricyclic antidepressants				
Amitriptyline	Major depression, dysthymia, obsessive-compulsive disorder, ADHD + tic disorders, Tourette's syndrome, separation anxiety, social phobia, enuresis	10–25 qhs	2–5	qhs–bid
Clomipramine				
Desipramine				
Imipramine				
Protriptyline				
Nortriptyline		10 qhs	1–3	qhs–bid

When the pediatrician lacks sufficient time to provide the necessary assessments, has limited expertise with these youth, or when suicidal ideation is present, referral or consultation is indicated.

Important factors in selection of a specific medication include relative safety for the particular patient, other medical conditions, comorbid psychiatric diagnoses, and suicide risk. The adolescent and parents should be familiarized with the risks and benefits of the medication, available alternative treatments, and possible adverse events. In addition, families should be informed that commonly used psychotropics often are not formally approved by the Food and Drug Administration for adolescents. Parents should administer and monitor the daily use of antidepressants in their children.

The promising research outcomes and tolerability of the SRIs make them the first-line agents for depressed adolescents. Although only the TCA and SRI antidepressants have been examined in controlled trials, other agents have been effective in adults and may benefit adolescents.

SEROTONIN REUPTAKE INHIBITORS

For depressed adolescents, SRIs are recommended because they appear efficacious; have few anticholinergic, sedative, or cardiovascular side effects; and are relatively safe with overdose. No physiologic or blood monitoring is necessary, and SRIs can be combined safely with other agents such as the stimulants when comorbid disorders such as ADHD are present.[10]

SRIs include fluoxetine (Prozac), sertraline (Zoloft), paroxetine (Paxil), fluvoxamine (Luvox), and venlafaxine (Effexor). Doses for adolescents approximate those used in adults. Common adverse effects include agitation, insomnia, nausea, weight loss, decreased libido, and irritability. Fluoxetine has a longer half-life than paroxetine or sertraline, possibly impeding resolution of the acute manic symptoms in "switching" adolescents. Fluvoxamine is more sedating, making it useful for children with sleep difficulties. Venlafaxine is a unique SRI with prominent noradrenergic properties, and it has been effective in refractory adult depression and in open studies of juveniles with depression or ADHD. All of these SRIs inhibit specific hepatic isoenzymes, potentially increasing levels of other medications, such as terfenadine.

Trazodone (Desyrel) and nefazodone (Serzone) also predominantly affect serotonin but at different receptor sites, resulting in different side effects than the traditional SRIs. These agents have been used less often for treating juvenile depression and are not generally considered first-line antidepressants.

ATYPICAL ANTIDEPRESSANTS

Bupropion (Wellbutrin) may be a first- or second-line agent in adolescents with (1) unstable mood such as depression in bipolar disorder or (2) depression plus ADHD. No controlled studies have been performed in depressed adolescents, but adult studies support its use in depression, ADHD, and possibly smoking cessation. Bupropion reduces the seizure threshold, particularly in high doses (6 mg/kg/d). Because bupropion may exacerbate tics, patients with tics should be closely monitored. A sustained-release preparation recently became available, allowing once or twice daily dosing and enhancing compliance.

Mirtazapine (Remeron) has noradrenergic and serotonergic properties, and recently has become available for adult depression. Clinical data in younger populations are not available, relegating this agent to use in juvenile depression refractory to the other agents.

Monoamine oxidase inhibitors (MAOIs) such as pargyline and tranylcypromine (Parnate) possess prominent, potentially harmful side effects and are not recommended for treatment of depressed adolescents. Specifically, MAOI-diet restrictions on cheeses, pizza, and other foods that are popular with adolescents dissuade use of these agents.

TRICYCLIC ANTIDEPRESSANTS

The TCAs are considered second-line agents for depressed adolescents. TCAs used in adolescents include amitriptyline (Elavil), imipramine (Tofranil), desipramine (Norpramin), and nortriptyline (Pamelor, Aventyl). These agents have varying affinities for norepinephrine and serotonin receptors, resulting in different side effect profiles. Approximately 5–10% of the population are "slow hydroxylators" (metabolizers) of TCAs, resulting in increased serum levels and warranting periodic serum measurements. Sudden cardiac death has been described in children receiving TCAs, but the risk for this does not appear significantly greater than in unmedicated children. TCA treatment should be preceded by a baseline EKG, and cardiac consultation is suggested for children with documented congenital or acquired cardiac disease, rhythm disturbances, or family history of premature cardiac disease. The recent American Academy of Pediatrics guidelines do not suggest routine EKG monitoring with TCAs, and guidelines for initiating and monitoring TCA treatment in adolescents have been described by Wilens et al.[31]

Common adverse effects of TCAs include anticholinergic effects of headaches, stomachaches, blurred vision, constipation, and dry mouth, which promotes tooth decay. TCAs can be fatal in overdose. To avoid withdrawal symptoms, tapering is recommended.

MANAGEMENT OF DEPRESSED ADOLESCENTS

Several guidelines may be used to enhance the adolescent's response to treatment. If no improvement occurs after 4 weeks on an adequate antidepressant dose, another agent should be considered.[25] If a mild response occurs by 4 weeks, continuation for 10 weeks may be required to optimize improvement.[2] Literature concerning adults suggests switching from one SRI to another rather than changing medication class when the first agent is ineffective.[4] Lithium augmentation may be helpful in depressed adolescents with prominent mood lability.[26] If the patient is refractory to two treatments or continues to deteriorate, mental health consultation is strongly encouraged.

Family members often inquire how long the adolescent should remain on antidepressant medication. Adolescents responsive to antidepressants should be maintained on medication for 6–12 months and symptom-free for at least 3 months before starting a slow downward titration of the medication (e.g., decreasing fluoxetine or paroxetine by 5–10 mg per week or decreasing sertraline by 12.5–25 mg per week). Monitoring the child for emergence of mood symptoms even when medication has been discontinued is necessary, because 40% may relapse within 2 years.[13] Reviewing past symptom progression and discussing reinstitution of treatment if 1–2 weeks of depressive symptoms return may reduce impairment from relapse. Because depression can be chronic, some adolescents may need to be maintained indefinitely on antidepressants.

CARING FOR BIPOLAR ADOLESCENTS

Bipolar disorder is among the most pernicious psychiatric disorders in youth. Although the pediatrician may not be primarily responsible for bipolar adolescents' medications, awareness of their pharmacologic principles may be helpful in the care of these patients. The primary mood-stabilizing agents are summarized in Table 4.

Response rates of adolescents to lithium (Eskalith, Lithobid) vacillate between 50–60%, about 20% lower than the response rate reported among adults, although bipolar adolescents treated with lithium are five times more likely to improve than youth receiving antidepressants, stimulants, neuroleptics, or anxiolytics.[3] Evidence suggests that alternative agents such as valproate (Depakene, Depakote) and carbamazepine (Tegretol) may be effective, first-line alternatives to lithium, in bipolar adolescents.[30]

Among the most troubling issues confronting anyone engaged in the longer term care of bipolar patients, particularly adolescents, is how to encourage compliance. About one-third of bipolar adolescents are noncompliant, and most noncompliant patients relapse.[28] Strategies to facilitate compliance in mood-disordered adolescents include frequent discussions about their disorder, close attention to side effects, and collaborating with adolescents to identify progressions of their symptoms and understand which medications address particular symptoms.

TABLE 4. Mood Stabilizers Used with Adolescents

Agent	Psychiatric Indications	Dosing (mg/kg/day)	Serum Level	Side Effects	Special Considerations
Lithium (Lithobid, Eskalith)	Bipolar disorder Depression Augmentation	10–30	0.5–1.4	Nausea, sedation, cognitive blunting, diarrhea, weight gain, psoriasis, acne	Low therapeutic ratio
Valproate (Depakote, Depakene)	Bipolar disorder	15–60	50–125	Nausea, headache, alopecia	Transient elevations in liver function tests may occur
Carbamazepine (Tegretol)	Bipolar disorder	10–20	4–12	Nausea, sedation, Stevens-Johnson syndrome, bone marrow suppression	Autoinduction may require increasing dose after 1–2 mo

SUMMARY

Mood disorders afflict pediatric patients, cause significant impairment, and interfere with normal adolescent development. Increasingly, pediatricians are called on to assess and collaborate with mental health practitioners in medicating adolescents with mood disorders. Approaching the adolescent with a primary emphasis on clarifying the diagnoses, determining environmental antecedents and sequelae, and investigating suicide risk enables the pediatrician to institute appropriate treatment. Although limited data from controlled studies exist in this population, the current practice is to prescribe psychotherapy as an initial treatment for mild to moderate depressions. Pharmacotherapy is supported in conjunction with psychotherapy in cases unresponsive to psychotherapy and in severe or suicidal cases. First-line pharmacotherapy for depressed adolescents is usually an SRI, followed by the atypical or TCA antidepressants. Bipolar disorder typically requires an aggressive medication regimen and environmental modifications. With severe, difficult, or refractory cases, mental health consultation is recommended to clarify diagnoses and to provide psychotherapy and input regarding medication.

References

1. Alpert JE, Maddocks A, Rosenbaum JF, Fava M: Childhood psychopathology retrospectively assessed among adults with early onset major depression. J Affect Disord 31:165–171, 1994.
2. Ambrosini PJ, Bianch MD, Metz C, Rabinovich H: Evaluating clinical response of open nortriptyline pharmacotherapy in adolescent major depression. J Child Adolesc Psychopharmacol 4:233–244, 1994.
3. Bostic JQ, Biederman J, Prince J, et al: Treatment course and outcome in children and adolescents diagnosed with mania by structured interview. Presented at the Annual Meeting of the American Academy of Child and Adolescent Psychiatry, Philadelphia, 1996.
4. Bostic JQ, Wilens, TE: Childhood mood disorders and office psychopharmacology. Pediatr Clin North Am (in press).
5. Bowden CL, Rhodes LJ: Mania in children and adolescents: Recognition and treatment. Psychiatr Ann 26 (Suppl):430–434, 1996.
6. Brent DA, Perper JA, Moritz G, et al: Psychiatric risk factors for adolescent suicide: A case-control study. J Am Acad Child Adolesc Psychiatry 32:521–529, 1993.
7. DSM-IV, Primary Care. Washington, DC, American Psychiatric Press, 1995.
8. Emslie GJ, Rush AJ, Weinberg WA, et al:A double-blind, randomized placebo-controlled trial of fluoxetine in depressed children and adolescents. Arch Gen Psychiatry (in press).
9. Fonagy P, Target M: Predictors of outcome in child psychoanalysis: A retrospective study of 763 cases at the Anna Freud Centre. J Am Psychoanal Assoc 44:27–77, 1996.
10. Gammon GD, Brown TE: Fluoxetine and methylphenidate in combination for treatment of attention deficit disorder and comorbid depressive disorder. J Child Adolesc Psychopharmacol 3:1–10, 1993.
11. Geller B, Cooper T, Graham D, et al: Double-blind placebo-controlled study of nortriptyline in depressed adolescents using a "fixed plasma level" design. Psychopharmacol Bull 26:85–90, 1990.
12 Geller B, Fox LW, Clark KA: Rate and predictors of prepubertal bipolarity during follow-up of 6- to 12-year-old children. J Am Acad Child Adolesc Psychiatry 33:461–468, 1994.
13. Hughes DC, Preskorn SH, Wrona M, et al: Follow up of adolescents initially treated for prepubertal-onset major depressive disorder with imipramine. Psychopharmacol Bull 26:244–248, 1990.
14. Kaminski KM, Naylor MW, King CA, Ghazuiddin N: Reactive mood and atypical depression in psychiatrically hospitalized depressed adolescents. Depression 3:176–181, 1995.
15. Koplewicz H, Klein R: Desipramine treatment in adolescent depression. Child Depression Consortium Meeting, Pittsburgh, PA, 1990.
16. Kovacs M: Presentation and course of major depressive disorder during childhood and later years of the life span. J Am Acad Child Adolesc Psychiatry 35:705–715, 1996.
17. Kramer AD, Feiguine RJ: Clinical effects of amitriptyline in adolescent depression. J Am Acad Child Adolesc Psychiatry 20:636–644, 1981.
18. Kutcher S, Boulos C, Ward B, et al: Response to desipramine treatment in adolescent depression: A fixed-dose, placebo-controlled trial. J Am Acad Child Adolesc Psychiatry 33:686–694, 1994.
19. Kye C, Waterman GS, Ryan ND, et al: A randomized, controlled trial of amitriptyline in the acute treatment of adolescent major depression. J Am Acad Child Adolesc Psychiatry 35:1139–1144, 1996.

20. Lewinsohn PM, Klein DN, Seeley JR: Bipolar disorders in a community sample of older adolescents: Prevalence, phenomenology, comorbidity, and course. J Am Acad Child Adolesc Psychiatry 34:454–463, 1995.
21. Pandey G: Platelet serotonin-2A receptors: A potential biological marker for suicidal behavior. Am J Psychiatry 152:850–855, 1995.
22. Pfeffer CR, Klerman GL, Hurt SW, et al: Suicidal children grow up: Rates and psychosocial risk factors for suicide attempts during follow-up. J Am Acad Child Adolesc Psychiatry 32:106–113, 1993.
23. Puig-Antich J, Luken E, Davies M, et al: Psychosocial functioning in prepubertal major depressive disorders: II. Arch Gen Psychiatry 42:511–517, 1985.
24. Puig-Antich J, Weston B: The diagnosis and treatment of major depressive disorder in childhood. Ann Rev Med 34:231–245, 1983.
25. Quitkin FM, McGrath PJ, Stewart, JW, et al: Chronological milestones to guide drug change. When should clinicians switch antidepressants? Arch Gen Psychiatry 53:785–792, 1996.
26. Ryan ND, Meyer V, Dachille S, et al: Lithium antidepressant augmentation in TCA-refractory depression in adolescents. J Am Acad Child Adolesc Psychiatry 27:371–376, 1988.
27. Simeon J, Dinicola V, Ferguson H, Copping W: Adolescent depression: a placebo-controlled fluoxetine treatment study and follow-up. Prog Neuropsychopharmacol Biol Psychiatry 14:791–795, 1990.
28. Strober M, Morrell W, Lampert C, et al: Relapse following discontinuation of lithium maintenance therapy in adolescents with bipolar I illness: A naturalistic study. Am J Psychiatry 147:457–461, 1990.
29. Weller RA, Kapadia P, Weller EB, et al: Psychopathology in families of children with major depressive disorders. J Affect Disord 31:247–252, 1994.
30. West SA, Keck PE, McElroy SL, et al: Open trial of valproate in the treatment of adolescent mania. J Child Adolesc Psychopharmacol 4:263–267, 1994.
31. Wilens TE, Biederman J, Baldessarini RJ, et al: Cardiovascular effects of therapeutic doses of tricyclic antidepressants in children and adolescents. J Am Acad Child Adolesc Psychiatry 35:1491–1501, 1996.
32. Wise N: In Their Own Words: Kurt Cobain & Courtney Love. New York, Omnibus, 1996.
33. Wozniak J, Biederman J, Kiely K, et al: Mania-like symptoms suggestive of childhood-onset bipolar disorder in clinically referred children. J Am Acad Child Adolesc Psychiatry 34:867–876, 1995.

Growth Hormone Treatment for Children without Growth Hormone Deficiency:

Does It Work and Will It Produce Adolescents Who Are Better Adjusted?

PAUL SAENGER, M.D.

Department of Pediatrics
Division of Pediatric Endocrinology
Albert Einstein College of Medicine/Montefiore Medical Center
Bronx, New York

Reprint requests to:
Paul Saenger, M.D.
Head, Division of Pediatric Endocrinology
Montefiore Medical Center
111 East 210th Street
Bronx, NY 10467

With the advent of recombinant DNA-generated growth hormone in 1985, the opportunities to treat children with organic or idiopathic growth hormone (GH) deficiencies are now, for the first time, unlimited. However, it has also become possible to treat short children who are not GH-deficient, and the selection of patients and effects of such treatment are only now being elucidated. Children with GH deficiency are typically below the fifth percentile in height, growth velocity is more than 2 standard deviations below age-appropriate norms, and their predicted adult height is significantly shorter than average. Children with organic GH deficiency, e.g., after removal of a pituitary tumor, may still be within the normal range for height, but growth velocity is distinctly abnormal. The unifying biochemical finding for these children is that they are found to be GH-deficient by a series of tests for pituitary GH secretion.

All of the tests for GH secretion share the problems of being expensive, having some degree of risk, having a strong dependence on the presence or absence of sex steroids (estrogens prime for growth hormone release), and lacking a clean separation of normal and abnormal growth hormone levels. Because different growth hormone assays on identical specimens give results with considerable variability, the determination of whether a patient could be considered GH-deficient depends on which assay was used. Furthermore, the coefficient of variation of repeated tests of stimulated or endogenous GH secretion is such that it is quite possible that the diagnosis of GH deficiency in a patient with short stature is more a matter of chance than science. It is not surprising, therefore, that many children with significant short stature who passed the test for growth hormone deficiency share the same clinical findings of short children diagnosed as growth hormone-deficient based on stimulation tests.

The health care provider, therefore, has to make an important decision at the outset of the evaluation of a child with short stature. The question is not so much how to test but rather whom to test for growth hormone adequacy. Documentation of clinical criteria is paramount for this decision. A child who is growing normally and has a height at or above the fifth percentile in most instances should not even be tested for growth hormone secretion and certainly should not be treated. GH is currently approved by the Food and Drug Administration only for the indications of GH deficiency, Turner syndrome, and short stature associated with chronic renal insufficiency. Use for idiopathic short stature (ISS), therefore, is an off-label use. This chapter discusses the use of recombinant DNA-generated GH for treatment of idiopathic short stature, Turner syndrome, and endstage renal disease. In addition, the psychologic effects of short stature and of treatment with GH are discussed.

IDIOPATHIC SHORT STATURE

Children with significant short stature (height below the fifth percentile) who do not have GH deficiency defined by classic criteria (GH above 10 ng/ml) are commonly referred to as having ISS and frequently seek treatment with GH. A series of studies detailed below describe the effect of GH in a group of children who are short and have a normal GH response to stimuli but have an abnormally slow growth velocity.

Another group commonly considered for GH therapy are children who are short, have a growth velocity appropriate for a child growing along or parallel to the fifth height percentile, and peak serum GH concentration that is also in the normal range. This group is most often referred to as having constitutional growth delay and short stature, familial short stature, or a combination of the two. Characteristically, those who have constitutional short stature also have a delayed bone age, whereas those who have familial short stature have normal bone ages and short parents.

Research confirms that these short children also respond to exogenous GH but their response is less than in those with classic GH deficiency and the therapeutic response often wanes after the first 2–3 years. In addition, there are some disturbing reports that GH treatment may actually accelerate the onset or progression of puberty, resulting in earlier cessation of growth and thus counteracting the desired treatment effects.

Evaluation and Treatment

Following recognition of the need for GH therapy for children who are definitely deficient in GH, the next therapeutic question is: What do we have to offer children who are short and who, following stimulatory tests, do not have definite GH deficiency? This is a difficult issue to resolve. In addition to the known limitations of radioimmunoassay measurements described above, it is possible that testing to provoke GH secretion frequently does not reflect endogenous GH secretion. Several groups who have used serial GH sampling techniques during 12-hour and 24-hour periods have shown a discrepancy between pharmacologic testing and spontaneous GH secretion in children who are short.[12] The term *neurosecretory dysfunction* was used initially to describe this entity, because some patients diagnosed as having neurosecretory dysfunction had received cranial radiation for the treatment of systemic or head and neck malignancies. It is well known that ionizing radiation of 24 Gy or more will dampen GH output. A recent study showed, however, that healthy children of normal height and children of idiopathic short stature may have the same low GH secretory profiles as those reported for patients who have organic hypothalamic-pituitary damage following irradiation. From these studies we may conclude that the physiologic approach of sampling GH every 20 minutes for 12 or 24 hours is no more sensitive than provocative tests in the detection of subtle forms of GH deficiency.[1]

Accordingly, the routine measurement of spontaneous GH secretion throughout 12 or 24 hours in the diagnosis of GH deficiency is not indicated. Although, in the case of healthy children, a positive correlation exists between profiles of GH secretion (as determined by frequent blood sampling techniques) and both height and height velocity, the range of overlap is large and does not allow a meaningful and reliable classification of individual patients. Because of the limited use of multiple sample testing, this technique must be relegated to the research environment. Rather, together with clinical assessment, measurements of components of the endocrine growth axis, i.e., insulin-like growth factor-1 (IGF-1), IGF binding protein-3 (IGFBP-3), *and* GH in response to provocative tests may allow a more meaningful assessment of "IGF deficiency."[14]

Admittedly, no convincing evidence supports the premise of a somatic disease in healthy children who are at either extreme of the normal distribution curve for height. In children who are short, evidence of psychologic impairment is tenuous at best, although numerous psychologic aspects of adolescence may be related to stature and the timing of sexual development.[2]

In the best of all possible worlds, the most effective response to "heightism" is a concerted effort to reveal and rectify height prejudice and not to accede to the demand for unrestricted use of GH. Unfortunately, sympathetic reassurance will satisfy only some parents, and well-intentioned counseling reinforcing the broad boundaries of normality is not successful with all families.

The rationale for an ongoing clinical trial detailed below is based on evidence from several studies that suggests that children with normal results on provocative testing of GH secretion may have short-term increases in their growth rate when given supplemental GH.

The best evidence that growth hormone therapy should be able to cause virtually any child to grow more rapidly and to attain a greater adult height lies in the observation that children with growth hormone-secreting pituitary tumors grow to be giants. The real questions do not relate to the efficacy of growth hormone but rather to whether increased adult height can be achieved with safe doses of growth hormone and whether such therapy is ethically justifiable and represents a suitable use of finite medical resources in an era dominated by aggressive cost containment.[13]

Preliminary Results of GH Treatment

Recently, 121 children with short stature who did not meet the classic criteria for GH deficiency were studied in a multicenter trial sponsored by Genentech, Inc and compared with an untreated control group.[6,7] The inclusion and exclusion criteria are shown in Table 1. Baseline characteristics (Table 2) were similar. As in most other studies, there was a marked male-over-female predominance. Also, the mean height of mothers and fathers was below average. Meaningful inspection of data required not only analysis of changes in growth rate but also of changes in predicted adult height in the treated group. Bone age advancement in the treated and untreated group was comparable. The growth rate can also be related to the rate of bone maturation by calculating the standard

TABLE 1. A Study of Idiopathic Short Stature: Inclusion and Exclusion Criteria

Inclusion Criteria	Exclusion Criteria
Age ≥ 5 years	Diabetes mellitus
Height ≤ 2 SD below mean for age (< 3rd percentile)	Hypothyroidism
Birth weight ≥ 2.5 kg	Any chronic systemic illness, including malignancy
Serum level of growth hormone of ≥ 10 ng/ml on at least one test	Any bone or cartilage dysplasia
Bone age: ≤ 9 years in girls, ≤ 10 years in boys	Psychosocial dwarfism
Prepubertal	Previous growth-promoting therapy
	Treatment for hyperactivity syndrome

From Hopwood NJ, Hintz RL, Gertner JM, et al: Growth response of non-growth hormone deficient children with marked short stature during three years of growth hormone therapy. J Pediatr 123:215, 1993, with permission.

deviation score (SDS) of height for bone age. The SDS is the difference between a patient's height (X) and mean normal height for the same bone age (x) divided by the standard deviation of height for that bone age. Thus, SDS = (X – x)/SD. In the study discussed, the SDS score increased in 1 year from –2.8 ± 0.9 to –2.2 ± 0 ($p < 0.00005$ compared with baseline).

These patients have now been treated for up to 9 years. Many have reached final height. GH therapy increased mean growth rate, height SDS, and Bayley-Pinneau predicted adult height (PAH) (Table 3). The mean difference between pretreatment PAH and final height was 4.9 ± 4.9 cm for males and 5.7 ± 5.2 cm for females. The average gain was +9.1 cm for males and 5.6 cm for females compared with untreated controls, and the expected mean final height increased by about 1 SD after GH therapy compared

TABLE 2. Baseline Characteristics of Patients in a Study of Idiopathic Short Stature

Characteristics*	Control Patients (n = 58)	Treatment Patients (n = 63)
Gender		
Male	43 (74%)	46 (73%)
Female	15 (26%)	17 (27%)
Age (y)	9.5 ± 2.4	9.4 ± 1.9
Bone age (y)	7.7 ± 2.3	7.9 ± 1.7
Age–bone age	1.8 ± 1.1	1.5 ± 1.0
Height (cm)	118.0 ± 11.2	118.0 ± 9.1
Height age (y)	6.5 ± 1.9	6.5 ± 1.5
Height (SD)	–2.8 ± 0.6	–2.7 ± 0.5
Weight (kg)	21.9 ± 5.1	22.1 ± 4.3
Prestudy growth rate (cm/y)	4.2 ± 1.2	4.6 ± 1.1
Mother's height (cm)†	156.5 ± 5.7	156.5 ± 6.3
Father's height (cm)§	170.7 ± 7.3	171.2 ± 8.0

*Values (except for gender) are expressed as mean ± standard deviation (SD).
All differences not significant ($p > 0.05$) on two-tailed t test.
† Normal mean = 163.7 ± 5.9.
§ Normal mean = 176.8 ± 6.5.
From Hopwood NJ, Hintz RL, Gertner JM, et al: Growth response of non-growth hormone deficient children with marked short stature during three years of growth hormone therapy. J Pediatr 123:215, 1993, with permission.

TABLE 3. Effect of Growth Hormone Treatment in Idiopathic Short Stature: Differences in Final Height and Predicted Adult Height (PAH)

			Change in Final Height/PAH (cm ± SD)		Change in Final Height/ Untreated Controls Who Were Short (≤ 2 SD)	
Study	**No.**	**Years of Therapy**	*Females (cm)*	*Males (cm)*	*Females (cm)*	*Males (cm)*
Hintz[6]	61	2–9	5.7 ± 5.2	4.9 ± 4.9	5.6	9.1
Loche[11]	15	4–10	None	None	Not done	
Hindmarsh[5]	9	4–9	2.5	2.8	Not done	
Kawai[8]	16 (only boys)	3.2–5	—	–8.6	Not done	

to untreated controls. Whether this beneficial effect is due to a correction of an abnormality of GH secretion or action, or due to pharmacologic effects of GH, remains to be determined. Mean final height, however, still was 0.5 SDS less than mean midparental target height.

Similar studies in a smaller group of children (n = 30) from the Netherlands obtained similar responses after 1 year of therapy.[21] When children had only a small height velocity increment after 1 year, the GH dosage was doubled, which was effective in increasing the growth velocity. The height velocity also remained significantly above baseline during the second year. Attenuation of the therapeutic response to GH is seen in both GH-deficient and non–GH-deficient children who are short. In published studies, administration of GH increased mean growth velocity by 2 cm per year in 75% of the treated healthy children who are short. The question remains whether GH may be useful for maximizing the height potential of healthy patients who are extremely short. The increase in growth velocity has not been as great as seen in classic GH deficiency, where a first-year response of 10.5 ± 2.2 cm per year commonly is seen with the same dosage of GH (0.3 mg/kg/week). This suggests that some patients who have idiopathic short stature may be less sensitive to GH treatment than patients who have severe GH deficiency.[10]

It is likely that children with heights 2 standard deviations below the mean may have been growing suboptimally (< 50th percentile of growth velocity for age) for several years. This conclusion is supported by the observation of the growth rate of the untreated control group in the Genentech study whose growth velocity did not change.

There were no significant anthropometric predictors of response, including bone age deficit or parental height. Little distinction was found between the responses of children classified as having familial short stature or constitutional short stature and the responses of the entire treatment population. This observation challenges the general belief that children who have familial short stature (those who commonly have little or no bone age delay and have short parents) are not likely to respond to exogenous growth hormone. Basal IGF-1 and IGFBP may correlate with GH responses to stimulation tests, but they do not aid in predicting who will respond to treatment. They do increase, however, with GH treatment and are useful to assess compliance with therapy.

Wit et al. argue that the absence of a consistent beneficial effect of GH treatment on height SDS for bone age, as seen in their study, should not be too disappointing.[21] Their findings are in concordance with long-term results for patients deficient in GH in whom height SDS for bone age did not change during GH therapy. The implication is that GH treatment cannot correct a deficit in height prognosis already present at diagnosis: it can only prevent further loss of stature and sometimes not even that.

Reporting on the long-term follow-up of untreated children with constitutional delay, La Franchi et al. found that boys were on average 5.1 cm and girls 5.3 cm under their target heights when remeasured as adults, compared with their predicted adult height.[9] We may conclude that many children with constitutional delay do not reach their genetic potential or that our methods of prediction are flawed.

After the initial enthusiasm for GH therapy in idiopathic short stature, fueled by optimistic results reported by Hopwood et al.,[7] there are now a number of reports that describe failures of growth hormone treatment to increase adult height in non–GH-deficient children with short stature. A small study by Kawai et al. published early this year found that in 18 short boys GH therapy was associated with earlier onset of puberty, briefer prepubertal duration, a significant decrease in height SDS for bone age during the pubertal period, and a resultant decrease in final height of almost 8 cm.[8]

Hindmarsh and Brook of Great Britain reported in 1996 that GH therapy significantly increased the final height of normal short children compared with their pretreatment predicted height, but this change was not significant compared with that observed in a small group of matched children without therapy.[5] A major part of the problem lies in the fact that most studies compare final height with predicted final height. Therapy with GH had no effect on the onset of puberty in this study, but treated boys progressed slightly faster through puberty than untreated boys, which was associated with an acceleration in bone age maturation. This acceleration in bone age maturation has a negative impact on final height, because closure of the epiphyses occurs sooner. In the view of the investigators, the small increment in final height—approximately 2.8 cm in boys and 2.5 cm in girls—does not justify the widespread use of GH for short children. Loche et al. also reported that the GH treatment of non–GH-deficient children resulted in a faster skeletal maturation and no significant improvement on the pretreatment predicted adult height.[11] In part, the disappointing results of some studies are due to the fact that the subject selection may have been less felicitous than desired. Normal short children who are growing at a near-normal growth rate may be less likely to show an accelerated growth velocity response after GH. On the other hand, normal short children with phenotypes most resembling those of GH-deficient children (poor growth rate, low IGF-1, low IGFBP-3, markedly delayed bone age, and height more than –2 SDS) may be more responsive.

The optimal dose of GH therapy remains unknown. While initial therapy may currently be adequate to stimulate growth rate as evidenced by rises in IGF-1, the dose may be inadequate to alter final height significantly, particularly since current treatment modalities do not foresee an increase in GH dosing during puberty, when physiologically robust increases in GH secretion and pulse amplitude occur. Hopwood et al., who reported the most optimistic results to date, found that children who remain prepubertal the longest had the greatest gain in height.[7] In this light it is interesting to note that the beneficial effect of GH on adult height reported in patients with Turner syndrome may be attributable, in part, to the failure of most girls with gonadal dysgenesis to enter puberty. This would then eliminate any potential effect of GH on early or rapid sexual maturation and thereby maximize its beneficial effect on stature.[14]

Partial GH insensitivity may be the cause for short stature in some patients.[4] A multicenter study to evaluate IGF-1 responses to GH treatment in ISS is underway in several centers. These studies will help to clarify the utility of IGF-1 measurements and IGF-1 response to GH treatment in honing our diagnostic abilities and predicting therapeutic response. According to Rosenfeld, this might sharpen our ability to distinguish normal children from those with underlying endocrine pathologic changes.[14] It is not likely that such additional tests would allow us unfailingly to diagnose children who would benefit from growth hormone treatment. While there may be a correlation between serum concentrations of IGF-1 and IGF-binding protein on provocative growth hormone tests, neither of the tests has been shown to be predictive of clinical responses to GH therapy. Therefore, the growth response during 1 year of treatment remains the gold standard to assess the efficacy of therapy.

We have not found any adverse effects on glucose metabolism or insulin levels in these long-term studies. Therapy did not alter serum electrolytes, lipids, thyroid hormone levels, and hemoglobin A_{1C}.[19] Blood pressure, plasma renin activity, and atrial natriuretic peptide also were not altered. Whether the use of drugs designed to delay puberty, such as gonadotropin-releasing hormone (GnRH) analogues, can be justified in this clinical setting remains to be determined.

GnRH analogues in combination with GH therapy might be beneficial. A potential side effect is decreased acquisition of bone mass, which typically occurs during adolescence. Alternatively, treatment with GnRH alone without GH has been shown to improve adult height in adolescents with short stature, as documented by preliminary results of a randomized, placebo-controlled trial.[3,22] The GnRH-treated group had a height gain over pretreatment predicted height of 6.2 ± 3.6 cm and an SDS gain over pretherapy predicted SDS of +1.1 ± 0.07.

While no final recommendations as far as therapeutic intervention with GH in normal short children can be offered, studies do suggest the potential efficacy in some children. These children show an acceleration in growth rate and a significant improvement in adult height. In normal short children, particularly those with normal growth velocities, therapy may lead to more rapid pubertal progression, negating any potential effect on adult height. GH treatment is certainly not indicated in the older short adolescent who has completed 95% of his or her growth. GH will simply not improve adult height. In the typical patient with constitutional delay of puberty and short stature and normal GH and IGF-1 levels, watchful waiting is best. If puberty is delayed beyond age 15 in boys, testosterone or oxandrolone is a safe, reasonable, and cheap therapeutic alternative.

TURNER SYNDROME

Short stature combined with a square appearance is the most common clinical feature of Turner syndrome. It is characterized by a tendency for mild intrauterine growth retardation (1 SD below the normal length at birth) as well as decreased growth rates during infancy and childhood and a pronounced lack of pubertal growth, resulting in a markedly reduced height of approximately 143 cm (56 in). Height should be plotted on growth curves specific for Turner syndrome. The final height of untreated patients correlates significantly with midparental height (r = 0.7).

The timely management of growth failure will affect many other aspects of Turner syndrome, including the age at which estrogen-replacement therapy should begin, socialization, and academic achievement. Since there is no growth hormone deficiency, provocative growth hormone testing need not be performed unless growth velocity is abnormal relative to that expected for Turner syndrome. Growth-promoting therapy with growth hormone alone or in combination with anabolic agents such as oxandrolone has become standard in many countries. Growth hormone therapy should be initiated as soon as the height of a girl with Turner syndrome drops below the fifth percentile of the normal female growth curve, which usually occurs at 2–5 years of age. Initially, growth hormone should be given at a dose of 0.05 mg per kilogram of body weight per day. In girls 9 to 12 years of age, combination therapy with growth hormone and an anabolic steroid (e.g,. oxandrolone at a dose of 0.0625 mg/kg/day) is recommended. Higher doses of oxandrolone may result in virilization and may hasten skeletal maturation. Therapy should be continued until the bone age exceeds 15 years and growth slows to less than 2 cm per year. Final heights well above 153 cm—a gain in predicted height of 10 cm—have been achieved in many treated patients. There is no rationale for estrogen therapy as a growth-promoting agent. In fact, in patients in whom estrogen therapy was initiated at or before 12 years of age, the degree of improvement in final height was significantly less (4–5 cm) than in those in whom therapy was started after 12 years of age. Poor outcomes are generally due to late initiation of growth hormone therapy and early estrogen therapy.

Other alternatives for growth promotion are orthopedic leg-lengthening procedures. These procedures are still possible after epiphyseal fusion has occurred. Experience with this approach in Turner syndrome is still limited.

Discussion with the patient and her family should help the physician decide when to initiate estrogen therapy to promote the development of secondary sex characteristics. I generally begin therapy when the girls are 14 years old, with excellent acceptance. Treatment should be with a natural estrogen, always beginning with a low daily dose, e.g., 0.3 mg of conjugated estrogens (Premarin), 0.5 mg of micronized estradiol (Estrace), or 0.3 mg of esterified estrogens (Menest or Estratab). The dose should gradually be increased to 1.25 mg in the case of conjugated estrogens so that feminization progresses gradually. This seems to produce better breast development than do maintenance doses of hormone-replacement therapy. Patients may think that breast development is suboptimal even after entirely appropriate estrogen-replacement therapy. This may be due in part to poor breast anlage, widely spaced nipples, and the shield chest. Adequate estrogen is essential to complete adolescent bone maturation, and estrogen requirements in these adolescent patients are therefore greater than those for older women treated with hormone-replacement therapy. Maintenance therapy should consist of 1.25 mg of conjugated estrogens per day. Progestin therapy, ideally with medroxyprogesterone acetate (Provera or Cycrin), is added for 12–14 days each month either when the first vaginal breakthrough bleeding occurs or in the second year of therapy. Once full pubertal maturation is achieved, many practitioners switch to a low-dose combination oral contraceptive pill, which is easier to take and promotes adherence to therapy.[16]

Slightly supraphysiologic doses of growth hormone are used in Turner syndrome. The same therapeutic approach has been successfully used in patients with endstage renal disease prior to transplantation.

CHILDREN WITH ENDSTAGE RENAL DISEASE

Patients who have uremia have normal to high GH secretion after provocation tests but show evidence for GH resistance (low free IGF-1). In short-term trials, this resistance has been overcome in most patients by supraphysiologic doses of GH. Initial data indicate that mean height velocity in uremic children nearly doubled without apparent significant side effects on carbohydrate metabolism or on renal function. Three-year successes again demonstrate the possibility of improving the growth velocity of children with chronic renal failure who are short, but it will be several years until data on adult height in these patients will become available.

After renal transplantation, children may show some short-lived improvement in growth velocity. However, children with transplants are typically on maintenance glucocorticoid therapy, which may impede growth. It has been demonstrated that growth hormone therapy in such children will overcome the potential adverse effects of glucocorticoid therapy. The question of an increase in rejection episodes while on growth hormone therapy after transplantation has not been completely answered. Although growth hormone therapy appears to be safe, it is not yet approved for posttransplantation treatment.

Use of recombinant DNA growth hormones in other conditions associated with short stature and normal growth hormone secretion such as Prader-Willi syndrome, Noonan's syndrome, inflammatory bowel disease, cystic fibrosis, and other chronic diseases associated with poor statural growth are experimental, and formal recommendations await the outcome of ongoing prospective clinical trials.

PSYCHOLOGIC EFFECTS OF SHORT STATURE

Reports on psychopathology associated with short stature are limited. An increased incidence of inattention and cognitive compromise in children who are deficient in GH but remain untreated has been described. Their inattention is not due to hyperactivity but to difficulties in short-term memory, concentration, and increased distractibility. In healthy children who are short and have heights around the fifth percentile, Cuttler et al. found normal psychosocial adaptation, and a full 48% of the children expressed satisfaction with their height.[2] In counseling parents and young patients, it is important to acknowledge and emphasize that there will always be a lowest fifth or tenth percentile and that this is normal.

Another important psychologic factor that must be considered is the effect on a child who is short if treatment with GH does not produce the desired increase in height. Even if certain children were not particularly self-conscious or worried about their height before treatment, the experience of a long series of painful injections may convince them that they have a serious disability. Thus, the treatment may plant the seeds of doubt and inferiority when, with parental acceptance and encouragement, they might never have existed.

In studies of psychologic effects of short stature in 11 children deficient in GH, Rotnem et al. reported: "Expectations of growth were heightened by elaborate endocrine evaluations and hospital admissions. These unrealized expectations contributed to the child's feeling that he was unacceptable as he was."[15] Further, as growth fell below parental expectations, the children "became acutely aware of the increased parental anxiety and disappointment, experiencing some of their parents' moods in themselves."[15] Until studies show that GH treatment improves psychosocial adjustment in non–GH-deficient children who are short, the use of GH cannot be justified by claiming that it provides psychosocial benefits.

If future clinical research shows that no psychosocial benefit accrues from treatment with GH, it should be acknowledged as a form of cosmetic therapy rather than treatment for a disease. Criteria for deciding when short stature is sufficiently deforming to warrant this form of therapy are needed to formulate rational and ethically acceptable criteria for hormonal therapy.[18]

There is only limited evidence that GH will make the healthy short patient a taller adult. Taller adult height should not be the a priori objective of therapy. Improved self-image and better psychosocial adjustment should be the decided objective. Otherwise we succumb to the hubris of heightism.

CONCLUSION

While GH treatment is of proven benefit in some non–GH-deficient patients with idiopathic short stature, the decision to use GH in idiopathic short stature is a complex issue that must involve accurate diagnosis of an abnormality in the GH/IGF axis and a candid discussion of the potential risks and benefits to the patient. In addition, the cost of treatment must be considered. One year of therapy may easily cost $25,000. Each millimeter in height gain may thus cost more than $1,000. These concerns only nourish our hope that oral nonpeptide GH secretagogues may be much cheaper once they are proven effective and approved for use in children.[17]

References

1. Bercu BB, Shulman D, Root AW, et al: Growth hormone provocative testing frequently does not reflect endogenous growth hormone secretion. J Clin Endocrinol Metab 63:709, 1986.
2. Cuttler L, Michon R, Reinecke M, Stocking C: Attitudinal and behavior concomitants of short stature. Pediatr Res 27:4A, 1990.
3. Gagne N, Van Vliet G, Blaquiere G, et al: GnRH analogues (GnRH-As) in combination with other hormone therapies in the management of short adolescents. Pediatr Res 39:89A, 1996.
4. Goddard AD, Cavello R, Luoh SM, et al, for the Growth Hormone Insensitivity Study Group: Mutations of the growth hormone receptor in children with idiopathic short stature. N Engl J Med 333:1093, 1995.
5. Hindmarsh PC, Brook CGD: Final height of short normal children treated with growth hormone. Lancet 348:13, 1996.
6. Hintz RL, Attie KM, Saenger P, et al: Growth hormone treatment of idiopathic short stature increases mean final height. N Engl J Med, in press.
7. Hopwood NJ, Hintz RL, Gertner JM, et al: Growth response of non-growth hormone deficient children with marked short stature during three years of growth hormone therapy. J Pediatr 123:215, 1993.
8. Kawai M, Momoi T, Yorifuji T, et al: Unfavorable effects of growth hormone therapy on the final height of boys with short stature not caused by growth hormone deficiency. J Pediatr 130:205, 1997.
9. LaFranchi S, Hanna CE, Mandel SH: Constitutional delay of growth: Expected vs. final adult height. Pediatrics 87:82, 1991.
10. Lesage C, Walker J, Landier F, et al: Near normalization of adolescent height with growth hormone therapy in very short children without growth hormone deficiency. J Pediatr 119:29, 1991.
11. Loche S, Cambiaso P, Setzu S, et al: Final height after growth hormone therapy in non-growth hormone-deficient children with short stature. J Pediatr 125:196, 1994.
12. Rose SR, Ross JL, Uriarte M, et al: The advantage of measuring stimulated as compared with spontaneous growth hormone levels in the diagnosis of growth hormone deficiency. N Engl J Med 319:201, 1988.
13. Rosenfeld RG: Editorial: Is growth hormone just a tall story? J Pediatr 130:172, 1997.
14. Rosenfeld RG, Albertsson-Wikland K, Cassorla F, et al: Diagnostic controversy: The diagnosis of childhood growth hormone deficiency: Revisited. J Clin Endocrinol Metab 80:1532, 1995.
15. Rotnem D, Cohen D, Hintz RL, et al: Psychological sequelae of relative treatment failure for children receiving human growth hormone replacement. J Am Acad Child Adolesc Psychiatry 18:505, 1979.
16. Saenger P: Current concepts: Turner's syndrome. N Engl J Med 335:1749, 1996.
17. Saenger P: Editorial: Oral growth hormones secretagogues—better than Alice in Wonderland's growth elixir. J Clin Endocrinol Metab 81:2773, 1996.
18. Saenger P: Use of growth hormone in the treatment of short stature: Boon or abuse. Pediatr Rev 12:355, 1991.
19. Saenger P, Attie KM, DiMartino-Nardi J, et al: Carbohydrate metabolism in children receiving growth hormone for 5 years. Pediatr Nephrol 10:261, 1996.
20. Toenshoff B, Mehls O, Heinrich U, et al: Growth-stimulating effects of recombinant human growth hormone in children with end stage renal disease. J Pediatr 116:561, 1990.
21. Wit JM, Fokker MH, de Muinck-Keizer-Schrama SMPF: Effects of two years of methionyl growth hormone in two dosage regimens in prepubertal children with short stature, subnormal growth rate and normal hormone response to secretagogues. J Pediatr 115:720, 1990.
22. Yanovski JA, Rose SR, Filmer KM, et al: Deslorelin-induced delay of puberty increases adult height of adolescents with short stature: Results of a randomized, placebo, controlled trial. Pediatr Res 39:101A, 1996.

Cosmetic Plastic Surgery in Adolescents

BERISH STRAUCH, M.D.
BRUCE GREENSTEIN, M.D.

Department of Plastic and Reconstructive Surgery
Albert Einstein College of Medicine and Montefiore Medical Center
Bronx, New York

Reprint requests to:
Berish Strauch, M.D.
Montefiore Medical Center
111 E. 210th Street
Bronx, NY 10470

ADOLESCENT PSYCHOLOGY AND PLASTIC SURGERY

Because of the adolescent's focus and emphasis on self-image, perceived or real physical deficits may be blamed for an inadequate sense of self and consequent social dysfunction or maladjustment. Plastic surgery procedures may be sought for corrections of defects and the achievement of a secure and positive self-identity. Functional indications such as nasal airway problems or dental malocclusion are usually fairly clear and readily identifiable. Psychosocial indications are more difficult to determine; however, failure to address them may lead to long-term consequences as severe and damaging as any functional problem.

An illustrative example is a port-wine stain of the cheek. Functionally, this is of little clinical significance other than it has a possible correlation with other birth defects. Skin with a port-wine stain does not have a greater incidence of infection, malignancy, or ulceration than the surrounding uninvolved skin. However, a port-wine stain may be clinically relevant in its psychological importance: it is a birthmark, an abnormality, something that makes the individual feel different and separate from others. Such patients may feel stigmatized to the point of believing that they can never be attractive or accepted. They may attempt to compensate for the birthmark or may avoid interpersonal contact. These reactions may represent alterations in behavior, but the functional significance of this skin vascular anomaly is simply that it exists.

Because the stain is visible, the example of a port-wine stain is relatively simple to comprehend.

Other "deformities"may be less obvious or not at all apparent to the outside observer. However, the psychosocial import of prominent ears, ethnic nose, or small breasts is quite significant: at issue are standards involving the adolescent's internalization of externally derived expectations. When these standards lead to a self-perceived lack, loss of self-esteem may follow. Such issues are salient in the struggle to establish an individual social identity apart from the family unit.

A primary goal of the plastic surgeon dealing with the adolescent patient should always be interaction with the patient, the family, and the primary physician (in addition to psychiatric or psychological counseling, when necessary) to determine if a surgical correction is warranted based on functional and/or psychosocial indications.

BREAST SURGERY

Historically, breasts have been symbols of femininity, fertility, and sexuality. Given this perspective, it is of little wonder that women in general and adolescent girls in particular frequently base a large amount of identity and self-esteem on the appearance of their breasts. "Perfect" breasts are amply displayed in the media and elsewhere, and the idealized breast has been defined most often by changing fashions. During the 1960s, relatively small breasts were the vogue, but more recent fashions have emphasized fuller breasts. An historical perspective, given these generalizations, may cause problems in the clinical management and indications for breast cosmetic surgery.

Hypomastia

Micromastia refers to an arrest in breast development in which lobule architecture develops but both the size and shape of the breasts remain juvenile. Hypomastia is a condition in which the breasts are judged by the patient and the clinician to be too small relative to the patient's body build. These conditions represent the most common developmental breast complaints. Small breasts may engender feelings of inadequacy that may lead to shy and withdrawn social behavior.

Infrequently, hypoplastic breast development may be asymmetric. Tuberous breasts may have an elongated shape and a constricted base, with most of the breast tissue located beneath the nipple-areola complex. In Poland's syndrome, there is partial or complete lack of growth of one breast, and there may be upper-limb abnormalities on the same side and complete or partial absence of the pectoral muscle ipsilaterally.

Surgery is generally considered following full physical maturation of the patient and stabilization of breast growth, usually not before a postmenarcheal age of 2–3 years. The surgical correction of hypomastia requires enlarging the breast mound, with breast augmentation usually accomplished by synthetic implants. Only in cases of Poland's syndrome, in which there is congenital absence of the pectoralis major muscle, does the surgeon consider using autogenous tissue. In addition to an implant, the latissimus dorsi muscle may be used to reconstruct the breast.

The use of implants for reconstruction or augmentation carries its own attendant problems. Given that the implant is not the patient's own tissue, the body develops a reaction to wall off the implant and creates a capsule surrounding the implant. Textured surfaces have been applied to implants to disturb the laminar nature of capsule formation and thus to prevent capsular contracture. Secondary procedures may be necessary if contracture becomes painful or otherwise symptomatic.

Saline-filled implants are common at present. When placed in a young patient, they are likely to eventually require replacement as a result of deflation.

Breast-implant augmentation has not been found to correlate with an increased incidence of human breast carcinoma. It does place greater technical demand on mammography technicians because, following augmentation, the breast mound is less compressible. Postaugmentation mammography requires multiview examinations so that as much of the breast as possible can be seen. Sonography and MRI are useful adjuncts to study the status and integrity of implants.

Breast augmentation is usually performed on an ambulatory basis, with the patient under local or general anesthesia. The breast implant may be placed beneath the breast tissue above the pectoralis or beneath the pectoralis major muscle. Subpectoral implants are recommended in patients with profound hypomastia because the implant is then placed beneath a greater volume of soft tissue.

Three types of incisions may be used for implant placement: periareolar, axillary, and inframammary. The periareolar incision is made at the junction of the inferior pole of the areola but is limited in its extent by the size of the areola itself (which should be at least 4 cm in diameter) and by the adjacent breast skin. The incision is well-camouflaged by the textured glandular nature of the areola. Axillary incisions are placed transversely in an axillary fold and are extremely well concealed. The limitations of the axillary approach arise from an inability to adequately develop the inferior pole of the implant pocket at the level of the inframammary crease; the use of the endoscope has facilitated this approach. Placement via an intraumbilical incision has been described, but many technical compromises are required with the use of this approach, and it has not become generally accepted. In addition, exposure and operative visualization are minimal. An inframammary approach provides direct access to the implant pocket, with the scar hidden in the inframammary crease or the undersurface of the breast.

Macromastia

Macromastia is characterized by breasts that are disproportionately large given the body habitus of the patient. Two clear clinical entities are virginal hypertrophic macromastia and symptomatic macromastia, the former usually blending with the latter.

In virginal hypertrophic macromastia, the breast parenchymal development induced by pubertal hormones is profound. The breasts are firm and large, tending toward gigantomastia. Patients complain of self-consciousness about excessive breast development and an inability to find clothes that adequately accommodate their breasts. They also report that social interactions are constrained by inappropriate attention to their breasts. Surgery is generally considered when no further growth of the breast has occurred for 1 year. However, intervention may become necessary if there is no cessation of breast growth and if the breasts are extremely large. Secondary procedures may be required should the breast continue to be oversized after a successful first operation.

Symptomatic macromastia arises from long-term postural compensation for excessive breast development. The patient's shoulders and upper back round and fail to support upper body weight. Complaints of chronic back pain, bra-strap grooving, and even symptoms of ulnar nerve compression may arise form postural compensation. Additionally, the patient may suffer from intertriginous infections of the inframammary crease secondary to macromastia. Patients with fully grown breasts that are stable in size and causative of symptoms are considered for reduction mammoplasty.

In some patients, the breast becomes severely ptotic due to involutional changes generally associated with weight changes and pregnancy. Correction will involve a procedure similar to that used for macromastia or using a prosthesis alone, with revision of the nipple-areola site.

Reduction mammoplasty procedures are based on preservation of the circulation and sensation to the nipple-areola complex whenever possible. Circulation can be maintained by basing the pedicle on the superior, lateral, or inferior circulation. The specific technique is selected based on the patient's attributes and the physician's preference.

Complications, although infrequent, may include hematoma, nipple loss, skin slough, infection, and scar hypertrophy. Breast sensitivity is generally retained after a reduction; however, in a few patients, sensitivity may be reduced and, rarely, totally absent. Depending on the extent of retention of the glandular duct system to the nipple, patients may be able to lactate, but the volume of milk may be significantly reduced. This is an important concern for the adolescent, who usually has not yet started her family, and must be addressed in presurgical counseling.

Gynecomastia

About 95% of cases of gynecomastia, the excessive development of male mammary glands, occur during puberty. Breast hypertrophy may be unilateral or bilateral. Most instances are related to increasing testosterone levels and will, to a large extent, involute over the course of several years. Gynecomastia has been associated with hypo- and hyperthyroidism, pituitary adenomas, acromegaly, juvenile cirrhosis, the use of marijuana and certain therapeutic medications, male pseudohermaphroditism, obesity, Klinefelter's syndrome, and testicular tumors, especially seminomas. The condition may also occur with the use of steroids by weightlifters.

Gynecomastia is of great concern to the affected adolescent male and, if left untreated, may result in significant psychological problems. The patient is embarrassed to undress in front of his peers in the locker room and usually will not engage in sports.

Preoperatively, careful examination of the breasts and testes is performed, and careful history and review of systems are obtained, with special emphasis on obtaining evidence of endocrinopathy. Endocrinologic consultation can rule out systemic abnormalities.

Once a decision is made to proceed with surgical correction, the nature of the scarring is discussed with the patient. For mild to moderate cases of gynecomastia, a periareolar incision is used and excess breast tissue removed. Liposuction has become a mainstay in cases of mild to moderate hypertrophy; it is often an adjunct procedure where direct excision is required. The resulting scar is well hidden in the junction of the pigmented nipple, areolar skin, and chest skin. A concentric circle technique resects skin circumferentially around the nipple, areola, and breast tissue, while nipple viability is maintained on a superior dermal pedicle; a circumferential scar around the areola results. Cases of significant skin excess will require horizontal and perhaps vertical chest scars that will be visible even after complete healing has occurred. The nipple may also be elevated using a minor variation of this technique. On occasion, drains may be needed postoperatively, and a compressive dressing is usually maintained over the chest for several days to minimize bleeding.

Although infrequent, complications are similar to those of reduction mammoplasty in the female: hematoma, nipple loss, skin slough, infection, and scar hypertrophy.

SUCTION LIPECTOMY

Suction lipectomy is a technique for body contouring, and the adolescent patient who is a candidate for this technique may enjoy maximal benefits. Youthful skin is more supple and better able to recontour following removal of localized areas of unsightly fat padding. However, suction lipectomy is not recommended for generalized weight loss. Its major indication is for local areas of excess fat distribution around the knee, trochanteric area, thighs, and abdomen; less frequently, the neck, ankle, and buttocks may be amenable to surgical correction. The adolescent need to look good in fashionable, tight-fitting clothes can sometimes be met by removal of discrete collections of adipose tissue.

The procedure may be performed under local or general anesthesia and may be done on an outpatient basis. Liposuction cannulas are introduced through small incisions near the area to be treated. Negative pressures just under 1 atm are generated. The cannulas are passed back and forth through the preoperatively marked areas, suctioning adipose tissue; the edges of the suctioned areas are feathered. Septae containing neurovascular structures are left intact, maintaining major nerves and vessels.

Most liposuction procedures are performed using a "tumescent" or "wet" technique. High volumes of very dilute local anesthetic and epinephrine solutions are infiltrated to allow for ease of fat removal and decrease of bleeding.

Postoperatively, the patient wears compression garments for several weeks. Autotransfusion is rarely required when large volumes of fat are removed. Untoward sequelae have been infrequent, with complications consisting of hypesthesia, seroma, edema formation and, to a lesser degree, hematomas, infections, and skin slough. There have been rare reports of fat emboli. Secondary procedures are possible.

LASER TREATMENT OF CUTANEOUS VASCULAR LESIONS

Benign vascular lesions such as telangiectasias, port-wine stains, and hemangiomas are of major concern to patients and parents, especially when they involve the face and other exposed areas of the body. The treatment of these lesions has been markedly improved by the use of tunable pulsed dye lasers. Selective photothermocoagulation of blood vessels occurs at a wavelength of 585 nm with the production of yellow light. Hemoglobin selectively absorbs yellow light, and thus the vessels differentially absorb the thermal energy. Minimal scarring results from laser treatment because of the minimal absorption of thermal energy at the dermal/epidermal junction.

With cooperative patients, the procedure may be performed with little discomfort; it often requires no anesthesia and can be done an on outpatient basis. Further advances in laser technology have broadened the applications in the treatment of other cutaneous lesions. Superficial pigmented lesions, as well as certain acne scars, may be treated with the CO_2 laser. Further future improvements in this technology are expected.

RHINOPLASTY

Rhinoplasty remains the most common aesthetic plastic surgery procedure in adolescents. The nose, because it constitutes the central element of the face, has enormous significance in the psychological and social domains. During adolescence, maturation of the face includes growth of the nose; under the influence of pubertal hormones, a cute childhood button nose may develop into a reflection of ethnic and genetic heritage. An adolescent whose self-image is largely externally derived may be unable successfully to incorporate a prominent nose or a large bump on the nose into a healthy self-perception.

A successful rhinoplasty can greatly enhance self-image; the change is quite clear to both the patient and others, and favorable external responses contribute greatly to a favorable outcome. Rhinoplasties can be performed in adolescents as young as 12, who are demonstrating no unusual growth of the nose with the onset of puberty and who already have a large nose with a projecting tip. However, the procedure, as well as all surgical corrections in adolescents, is best deferred until the completion of growth and maturation at Tanner stage 5. This delay eliminates the possibility of further growth and and development attenuating the postoperative outcome. Female nasal development is 90% complete by age 13–16 years, and male development by age 15–18. "Full development" refers to completion of the cartilaginous and bony architecture of the nose; changes in the integument continue throughout life.

Preoperatively, attentive listening to the patient remains the most important aspect of the examination. Complaints in excess of physical findings may indicate some psychological disturbance; in such cases, counseling is recommended. In addition, different ethnic groups have different aesthetic values, and a surgeon who ignores the patient's desire to follow some sort of surgical and aesthetic "ideal" may produce an outcome that is unacceptable. It is critically important to ask the patient for a specific description of the change desired in nasal appearance. Any airway obstruction should be evaluated preoperatively and concomitant septal or turbinate surgery can be performed, if required.

The current standard of beauty is a nose that is almost completely straight in profile except for the projection of the tip. Many consider the scooped-out, "ski-jump" nasal profile to be a deformity. The appearance of the nostrils must also be taken into consideration, because the patient may believe that wide, flaring nostrils require surgical correction.

Almost all adolescent rhinoplasties are performed with the patient under local anesthesia, combined with pre- and intraoperative administration of sedatives. Rhinoplasties are generally approached through intranasal or external incisions. Many procedures use a technique involving a small, external incision at the base of the columella so that an "open" rhinoplasty can be carried out. This technique allows for better visualization and sculpting of the nasal cartilage. If such areas of the nose as the dorsum or tip require augmentation, cartilage from the septum or, if necessary, from the ear, may be harvested. Major dorsal profile augmentation may require the use of tissues from other donor sites or autologous grafts such as irradiated rib cartilage grafts. Bone or cartilage grafts can be harvested from the calvarium, ribs, iliac crest, or ears.

All internal incisions are sutured with absorbable materials that do not require removal. The nose is then packed to prevent adhesion formation between the intranasal incisions. This packing is usually removed after 24–48 hours unless septal surgery has been performed. In the latter instance, packing remains in place longer. An external splint is worn for about a week to maintain the nasal bones in position. The patient is placed on a diet that requires minimal mastication and is discharged 24 hours after the procedure.

The most common postoperative complication is epistaxis. Bleeding may occur immediately postoperatively or at an interval of 10–14 days. Most bleeding can be treated with repeat packing. Infection after rhinoplasty is rare. Swelling of the nose after surgery is not unusual and may last for several weeks to months, especially swelling at the tip.

Following a technically successful rhinoplasty, most properly selected adolescents express satisfaction with the postoperative results, especially as they receive positive reinforcement about the change in their appearance from their peers and even themselves.

MENTOPLASTY

Optimal results of rhinoplasty can be obtained only if the chin position is in harmony with the rest of the face. The aesthetic balance between forehead, nose, and chin is of major importance. Major chin deformities are usually associated with dental occlusive abnormalities and require mandibular and perhaps maxillary surgery for correction.

Most patients with chin deformities are unaware of an abnormal profile beyond their expression of dissatisfaction with the appearance of the nose.

In these situations, the surgeon should carefully examine the position of the chin, which should project beyond a line drawn through the glabella and upper lip. Prognathism, or the prominence of the jaw in both full-face and profile views, may require treatment. Rarely, the chin alone may be excessively large, with a normal occlusive relationship, and this condition is considered true macrogenia. Preoperatively, cephalometric radiographs, the standard for measuring dental and facial proportions, may be helpful in determining how much correction is required.

For a retruded or small chin, two procedures are possible. In the most common approach, a Silastic implant is placed through an intraoral or submental incision while the patient is under local anesthesia. The implant is then supported with external taping to avoid displacement. The alternative procedure is a sliding genioplasty, which is repositioning of the chin by performing a horizontal osteotomy within the mandible. The chin can then be advanced by sliding the segment forward, or reduced by lowering the height, or retruded by sliding the segment backward. Internal wires or plates are used to maintain the corrected chin position. Immediately preoperatively, the patient is placed on a liquid diet, which is followed by a diet requiring minimal mastication.

Potential complications include hypesthesia resulting from injury to the inferior alveolar nerve. This problem rarely occurs with implants, and although more common with osteotomies, permanent severe alterations in sensibility remain rare. Hematoma is a rare postoperative problem. Infections are unusual, but they may necessitate removal of the implant or wires placed for the genioplasty. Extrusion of Silastic implants can occur, and secondary correction may be required.

CRANIOFACIAL SURGERY

The current philosophy in craniofacial surgery involves the notion that correction of any facial deformity requires that the facial skeleton be made anatomically normal. This simple concept has provided new possibilities in the correction of congenital craniofacial disorders. Prior to Tessier's work, most of these disorders were treated by camouflage procedures in which bone grafts were onlayed to the facial skeleton for augmenting bony deficits and filling in bony defects. Now, the challenge to the craniofacial surgeon is to restructure the abnormal facial skeleton by bringing the bones into normal anatomic relationships through the use of carefully placed osteotomies.

In the past, craniofacial procedures were performed in older adolescents and young adults; their ability to tolerate the length and magnitude of the operative procedure were believed to make them the best candidates for this surgery. As the techniques in craniofacial surgery have been refined, the age at which it can be performed has become progressively younger. However, psychosocial and physiologic considerations dictate the timing of craniofacial reconstruction, and adolescence and young adulthood remain the most ideal times for orbital and midfacial reconstruction. During late puberty, the facial skeleton undergoes final maturation; therefore, a surgical reconstruction will not destroy areas of active growth or be altered by unarrested growth processes.

Procedures performed by the craniofacial surgeon may be considered in three categories: orbitotomy, midfacial advancement, and mandibulotomy.

In orbitotomy, the orbital skeleton is separated from the cranium and maxilla to correct orbital dystopia and ocular hypertelorism. In the surgical correction of orbital dystopia, a C-osteotomy that includes the lateral portion of the superior orbital brow, lateral orbital wall, and inferior orbital rim is performed, and these structures are moved as a unit. The unit may be moved superiorly, laterally, or inferiorly to bring the bony orbital wall of one orbit into alignment with the anatomic position of the contralateral orbit. In the surgical correction of ocular hypertelorism, both orbits are operated on simultaneously. Osteotomies of the superior orbital wall, superior orbital rim, medial orbital walls, inferior orbital floors, and lateral orbital walls are performed so that each orbit constitutes a bony rectangle. The nasal ethmoid region is then resected, allowing these bony rectangles to be moved closer to the midline and thereby eliminating the increased intercanthal space.

Midfacial advancement is indicated when the patient has a clinical class III malocclusion in which the maxillary arch lies posterior to the mandibular arch and the position of the mandible is normal relative to the cranial base. Midfacial advancements can be performed at various levels. LeFort I advancement brings the alveolar segment of the maxilla with its definition forward, affecting only the tip and base of the nose. LeFort I midfacial advancement is frequently used for correction of mandibular/maxillary dental disharmony. The LeFort II procedure advances the nasal root and central pyramid of the maxilla, leaving the inferior orbital rims and zygomas of the face unaffected. The LeFort III midfacial advancement advances the entire maxilla, zygomas, and inferior orbital floors relative to the mandible and cranial base.

The LeFort II procedure is frequently performed for correction of posttraumatic facial deformities, and the LeFort III midfacial advancement is most often used for correction of congenital midfacial deficiencies, such as those demonstrated in Crouzon's, Apert's, and Pfeiffer syndromes.

Mandibulotomies are surgical osteotomies within the bony arch of the mandible. In craniofacial surgery, mandibular osteotomies are frequently limited to genioplasties, in which a horizontal mandibular osteotomy is used to advance or reduce the prominence of the chin.

Craniofacial surgery itself is a sub-area of plastic surgery that can create a semblance of the normal facial appearance even in the most severe congenital deformities. The procedures place great demands on the patient and physician; however, at their best, they can provide improved facial appearance, consequent patient confidence, and possible societal integration.

CONCLUSIONS

Adolescence is a period of awakening, a transition from childhood to adulthood. It may be a period of psychosocial instability, since it is during this time that the adolescent usually establishes a self-identity requiring separation from familial dependence and incorporation into a larger social network. During this transition period, insecurities and feelings of inadequacy may surface.

Since adolescent self-perception may be in a state of flux in any case, this inherent instability can produce profound self-doubt but can also produce rapid adaptation to changes in physical appearance—a plasticity of self-perception that works on behalf of the plastic surgeon.

References

1. Born G: The "L" mammoplasty. Ann Plast Surg 32:283, 1994.
2. Brink RR: Management of true ptosis of the breast. Plast Reconstr Surg 91:657, 1993.
3. de la Fuente A, Martin del Yerro JL: Periareolar mastopexy with mammary implants. Aesthet Plast Surg 16:337, 1992.
4. Flowers RS: Alloplastic augmentation of the anterior mandible. Clin Plast Surg 18:107, 1991.

5. Goin JM, Goin MK: Changing the Body: Psychological Effects of Plastic Surgery. Baltimore, Williams & Wilkins, 1986.
6. Goodrich JT, Poast KD, Argamaso RV: Plastic Techniques in Neurosurgery. New York, Thieme, 1991.
7. Juma A, Miller JG, Laitung JK: Pedicle deepithelialization in breast reduction and mastopexy using the electric dermatome [letter]. Plast Reconstr Surg 95:216, 1995.
8. Lejour M: Vertical mammoplasty and liposuction of the breast. Plast Reconstr Surg 94:100, 1994.
9. Martin del Yerro JL: Periareolar mastopexy with mammary implants. Aesthet Plast Surg 16:337, 1992.
10. McCarthy JG, Ruff GL, Zide BM: A surgical system for the correction of bony chin deformity. Clin Plast Surg 18:139, 1991.
11. Robbins LB, Hoffman DK: The superior dermoglandular pedicle approach to breast reduction. Ann Plast Surg 29:211, 1992.
12. Rose NR: Nonimmunogenicity of Silastic [letter]. In Additional Comments from Plastic Surgery to the FDA, prepared by members of the Silicone Implant Research Committee of the Plastic Surgery Educational Foundation, February 1991.
13. Sandsmark M, Amland PF, Samdal F, et al: Clinical results in 87 patients treated for asymmetrical breasts: A follow-up study. Scand J Plast Reconstr Surg Hand Surg 126:321, 1992.
14. Stambaugh KI: Chin augmentation: An important adjunctive procedure to rhinoplasty. Arch Otolaryngol Head Neck Surg 118:682, 1992.
15. Thomson HG: Common benign pediatric cutaneous tumors: Timing and treatment. Clin Plast Surg 17:55, 1990.
16. Whitaker LA: Aesthetic surgery of the facial skeleton. Clin Plast Surg 18:153, 1991.

Index

Entries in **boldface** type indicate complete chapters.